Ocean of Yoga

T0204833

of related interest

The Meditation Book of Light and Colour
Pauline Wills
ISBN 978 1 84819 202 7
eISBN 978 0 85701 162 6

Body Intelligence Meditation
Finding presence through embodiment
Ged Sumner
ISBN 978 1 84819 174 7
eISBN 978 0 85701 121 3

Mudras of Yoga
72 Hand Gestures for Healing and Spiritual Growth
Cain Carroll with Revital Carroll
ISBN 978 1 84819 176 1 (card set)
eISBN 978 0 85701 143 5

Ocean of
YOGA

Meditations on Yoga and Āyurveda for
Balance, Awareness, and Well-Being

Julie Dunlop

Foreword by Vasant Lad, B.A.M. & S., M.A.Sc.

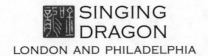

SINGING
DRAGON

LONDON AND PHILADELPHIA

First published in 2018
by Singing Dragon
an imprint of Jessica Kingsley Publishers
73 Collier Street
London N1 9BE, UK
and
400 Market Street, Suite 400
Philadelphia, PA 19106, USA

www.singingdragon.com

Library of Congress Cataloging in Publication Data
A CIP catalog record for this book is available from the Library of Congress

British Library Cataloguing in Publication Data
A CIP catalogue record for this book is available from the British Library

ISBN 978 1 84819 360 4
eISBN 978 0 85701 318 7

Printed and bound in the United States

This Book Is Dedicated…

To yoga, in all of its many forms

To Āyurveda—its beauty, its balance, its healing potency and grace

To all those who have carried the teachings and lineage of yoga and Āyurveda through the generations to arrive to us, today, here, now

To the *doṣhas*, *guṇas*, and *pañcha mahābhūtas* that comprise us and our world, as well as the prayers, *mantras*, *prāṇāyāmas*, and *āsanas* that support us in our daily well-being

To Vasant Lad, founder of the Ayurvedic Institute in Albuquerque, whose compassion, knowledge, kindness, wisdom, innovation, humor, and humility have inspired me daily since I first heard him speak in 2005; the weaving together of science, medicine, history, philosophy, art, poetry, stories, and music in his teaching is profound

To all of my teachers in yoga, in Āyurveda, in writing, and in life who have taught me more than I could measure, and to all of my students whose dedication to learning is an unending source of inspiration

To Grandmother, who, through the beautiful book of her daily life, shared tranquility, creativity, and integrity, and who, by welcoming me into her home in the mountains of Appalachia, blessed my life immensely

To Margaret ("M"), my dear four-footed one who loved to be near meditation, *prāṇāyāma*, and *āsana*, and whose patience, enthusiasm, intuition, authenticity, and unconditional love was and is a deeply healing presence in my life

To my parents, Karen and Jim Dunlop, for giving me the gift of life, and whose love, encouragement, understanding, and support humble me daily as my journey continues to unfold

To our ancestors, without whom we would not be here

And to you, reader, whose sacred presence brings the words of this book to life.

In Memory

This book is dedicated to the memory of:

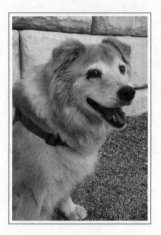

"M"
(Margaret)
circa 2000—July 8, 2016

Into the palpable presence of the absence of the four-footed yogini
who had been by my side for fifteen years came the words of this
book, arriving just as unexpectedly as she did back in 2001.

Yogis and yoginis come in many forms.

Contents

Foreword

The word "yoga" has become popular all over the world since Swāmī Vivekānanda, an innately loving, very compassionate disciple of Śrī Rāmakṛṣṇa Paramahamsa, came to the United States over a hundred years ago to attend an all-religions conference, and there he spoke about Vedanta and yoga philosophy. As we know, "yoga," coming from the word "*yuj*," means "to unite." It is an ancient art of union of the lower self with the higher self by following yogic discipline. Yoga is very ancient in India. Even before Patañjali's *Yoga Sūtras*, there were *rishis* all having their own names with the yoga; for example, the guru of Śrī Rām was Vasiṣṭha: Vasiṣṭha yoga. Vālmīki yoga, Sandīpanī yoga, Śāṇḍilya yoga, and Kaśyapa yoga: all these different *rishis* had their permutations and combinations in the unique system of yoga, and they developed their own system of enlightenment.

Aṣṭāṅga yoga is the eight limbs of yoga—*yama, niyama, āsana, prāṇāyāma, pratyāhāra, dhāraṇā, dhyāna, samādhi*. The first two *aṅga*, the first two limbs, *yama* and *niyama*, are a wonderful discipline, and that discipline is the foundation of the yoga system. Then comes *āsana*. *Āsana* is *sthira sukham āsanam*; one can sit in that posture without any pain, without any discomfort, without any effort. Such an effortless, quiet, peaceful, relaxing state of awareness is called *āsana*, and there are 8.4 million postures; I think out of 8.4 million, we should know 84. Out of 84, we should do at least eight *āsanas* in our daily life to keep our body, mind, and consciousness in harmony with the universal law. Yoga follows the universal law of perfect health.

My student Julie Dunlop's book reflects her dedication, devotion, and great commitment to the ancient yogic disciplines. This is definitely her lifetime work, and she has put it into wonderful poetry in constant, continuous flow of awareness under the name *Ocean of Yoga*. In the ocean, all rivers come and meet with the ocean; similarly, in this book, all different systems of yoga blend together in order to bring the radical healing of the body, mind, and consciousness.

This book, *Ocean of Yoga*, includes meditations on yoga and Āyurveda for balancing awareness and well-being. My loving, compassionate, dedicated student Julie Dunlop has learned the basic principles of Āyurveda by heart, and she has completed Ayurvedic Studies Program 1 and Ayurvedic Studies Program 2. From Julie Dunlop's great experience of Āyurveda and following yogic discipline, this book is an outcome of her effort, experience, dedication, and devotion; it is a very sacred work of integration of Āyurveda and yoga.

In this book, the endless, timeless wisdom of Āyurveda and yoga are beautifully woven together. She talks about walking along the shore, gratitude, the riding of the waves, the setting of intention, and she talks about heart, laughter, tears, and receiving the teachings. She also talks a great deal about the three *doṣhas* and how to bring them into harmony. Chapter by chapter, she has revealed the yogic discipline and Ayurvedic discipline. This is a great work of integration that Julie has done, and I truly admire this; it is a masterpiece of work of Julie's devotion. I'm quite sure that this book will help readers to bring Ayurvedic and yogic discipline to their lives, and I hope this book will help the reader to attain *samādhi*, the transcendental state of awareness. The secret meaning of yoga is "skill in action" (*yogaḥ karmasu kauśalam*). The reader will develop not only the skill in action but also the skill in daily life-relationship, which will make the life whole, and whole is holy.

Love and Light,
Vasant Lad, B.A.M. & S., M.A.Sc.
The Ayurvedic Institute
Albuquerque, New Mexico
May 2017

*May we infuse the wisdom of our practice
into
the moments of our lives*

Preface

Yoga, with its rich tradition of millennia, is as vast and deep as the ocean. When we go to the ocean and step in, perhaps even swim in the waves a bit, we feel we have been to the ocean—and we have—and yet, we have sampled only one tiny part of one of the many vast oceans of the world. Similarly, when we go to a yoga class, we become immersed within yoga— and yet it is just one day's practice out of a lifetime, and it is one style or lineage of yoga out of many; we have touched the ocean of yoga.

Yoga, while often understood to be the practice of *āsana* (physical postures) on a mat, extends well beyond this realm, flowing into every moment of our lives. In our fast-paced, electronically-stimulated world, it is easy to move away from, rather than towards, our own well-being, forgetting our center. Through the various challenges and stresses we face, we can temporarily lose touch with a balanced life, a balanced perspective. However, through awareness and meditative focus, both in our thoughts and actions, we can regain a sense of well-being. The eight limbs of yoga and the basic principles of yoga's sister science, Āyurveda, offer us many gems of wisdom that reflect the essence of light like ocean waves sparkling in the sun.

Introduction

The ocean of yoga can surprise us with what it washes up on our shore. That has certainly been the case for me. I share with you these meditations and reflections that I did not know would be coming until they began to arrive in the autumn of 2016. If, for you, they in any way hint at the depth and calm and power of yoga's ocean as you have experienced it, I am profoundly grateful, and if they do not, please let them drift back into the cosmic ocean to be further washed and purified by the divinity of transformation that exists in all things.

When we sit in *Baddha Koṇāsana* (Bound Angle) and gently open the inside edges of our feet, it is as if we are reading a small book. In the lines of the soles of our feet and in the invisible vestiges of the inches and miles they have traveled is the story of our individual lives and of life as a whole. A record of every place we have stood and every moment we have traversed in this life is present as we continue writing with the divine ink of each of our experiences, each day greeting us with beauty, challenges, and possibility.

This book, a drop in the ocean, is an offering of gratitude to yoga and Āyurveda for the many gifts and lessons they have brought and continue to bring, and to my teachers who, through their patience, skill, inspiration, and wisdom, have helped me in innumerable ways.

Ocean of Yoga comes forth from everyone and everything I have known in this life, all of the places, people, animals, conversations, silences, interactions, and experiences that have become a part of me, shaping me, teaching me, uplifting me, humbling me, and helping me grow.

To God and this divine life, I bow.

As We Begin...

- Thank you for your presence, for arriving here to this page, just as you are. You are an exquisite part of the ocean of breath and life, connecting us all in sacred community.

- The meditations in this collection are best read slowly, one at a time, silently or aloud, either in part or in full, perhaps in a yoga class, or as part of your personal practice.

- Just as the ocean cannot be crossed all at once, pace yourself as you read. You might start at the end, middle, or beginning, depending upon what you feel drawn to. The book begins with a collection of opening meditations that can be used at the start of a yoga class or at the start of an individual practice. The book then continues into a "Diving Deeper" section of yoga philosophy, contemplating the eight limbs of yoga, five obstacles that can interfere with our practice, and the seven *chakras* that grace our anatomical architecture. The next section, "Yoga's Sister Sea: Āyurveda," explores facets of Āyurveda, the ancient medical science from India, which shares yoga's focus of enhancing the well-being of body, mind, and soul. "The Ocean's Depths" offers a collection of guided meditations that can be read aloud during the resting period (*Shavāsana*) at the end of a yoga class or read silently to invite relaxation. Finally, there are closing meditations to seal the practice, either in a yoga class or on your own, as well as contemplations for reflection. Please take what works for you and let the rest drift back to sea.

- The meditations in this collection are interpretative and experiential. The experience of seeing sunlight on ocean waves is different, for instance, than a scientific study of the particles of water and light. For scholarly exploration of the eight limbs of yoga, *chakras*, and Āyurveda, many ancient Vedic texts as well as modern texts abound (the Bibliography and Related Resources sections at the end of the book offer some examples).

- Please note that the information and meditations in this book are not designed to diagnose or treat medical issues. If you have a medical concern, please consult with your physician or licensed health professional to receive individualized care.

- If you come across words that are unfamiliar to you, you may wish, for now, to simply pause and observe them as you might pick up shells to look at as you walk beside the sea.

- Traditional Sanskrit terms (along with translations) have been included to honor the vibration of the original language of Yoga and Āyurveda.

  Note: In the case of **c**, **ch** has been substituted; also, in the case of ṣ, **ṣh** has been substituted, and in the case of ś, **sh** has been used to assist with ease of pronunciation for those not familiar with Sanskrit.

- Thank you for your shining presence.
  May we always remember the light that we carry within.

One Page, One Breath at a Time

This book is about slowing down, not speeding up. It is about taking time to notice—the movement of breath through your body, the movement of wind through the trees, the movement of feelings and thoughts circulating through you. It is about noticing—and welcoming—stillness, silence, peace, balance, and well-being.

To receive the maximum benefit in reading this book, pause for a few minutes after reading each page.

One possible path is to read an opening meditation and begin your practice. Another path is to begin your practice and finish with a closing meditation. Or you might read other sections when you are not able to practice.

The meditations can be read in any order. The section on Āyurveda, however, may be most effectively digested when read sequentially.

Reading meditations meditatively, rather than in a hurry, invites awareness and a deepening of the practice. Reading the book all at once, or even one section all at once, might be a little like ordering one of every item on a menu. Instead of taxing the digestive system of the mind, allow yourself to enjoy, sampling one page per day or one page per practice, or at a pace that works well for you.

So go slowly, if you can, and if you can't, notice that, too. Just as we renew ourselves each time we return to the mat, we are new each time we continue, whether it is returning to a book, a situation, a location, a conversation, or meditation.

ॐ Dear Reader

Dear Reader, you who are arriving here
by intuition, volition, or some unknown path

you, with your eyes shining
like two luminous globes,

you with your heart open
like a savannah
or shut tight
like a locked vault

you, with your memories, joys, griefs,
and consternations
glowing like constellations
in a cosmos vastly brilliant
beneath your humble skull

you, with the lobes of your lungs
breathing in tandem
in the most magnificent duet
of the symphony
playing on even as you sleep

you with your network of nerves
putting the fastest Wi-Fi to shame,
the exquisite ladder of your spine
holding your head erect
showcasing the singular flower
of your face

you with your inclinations and hesitations,
with your inspirations, contemplations, and frustrations,
with your practice and presence,
your humility, wisdom, and grace,
your resistance and resilience,

I say, without equivocation, reservation, or deliberation,
you, with utmost dedication,
are yoga—the vastness, depth, and beauty of its ocean,
composite of infinite individual waves.

WALKING ALONG THE SHORE
Opening Meditations

....

Beginning a yoga practice with meditation can help us to pause and center as we transition from whatever we were doing—driving, walking, texting, talking, or something else—before arriving at our mat.

ॐ Gratitude

You are here. Thank you. The fact that you made space and time in your day to be here is significant. Maybe you almost didn't show up. Maybe you were running late. Maybe you are feeling really well, and then again, maybe you are not. Maybe you are feeling tired. Maybe you have aches and pains. Maybe something is weighing on your heart. Breathe.

You are here. Breathe. Feel what you feel—in your body, in your mind, in your soul. Placing your hands at your heart, thank yourself for being here. If you feel so led, you may wish to offer gratitude to those people and circumstances that are allowing your practice to take place today.

Strengthening and renewing ourselves through our practice is a way to give thanks for this life we are living and to put ourselves in a better position to have the energy to help and serve others.

Breathe in, opening yourself to receiving. Breathe out, letting go of any holding.

Is your body here? Is your mind here? Is your soul here?

Enter into the space of you, the space of this room, this practice as fully as you can.

You are here. Feel the rise and fall of your chest where the heart sings.

ॐ Riding the Waves

O ne of yoga's gifts is teaching us to be present. While this may seem like it should come naturally, and perhaps it did for many of our ancestors in years past, today's culture, in many places, tends to gravitate towards fragmentation and rushing, rather than a focused, calm stillness. The choice is ours. We can resist and struggle, flailing, flapping our arms, exhausting ourselves as we try to tread water in the deep seas of life—or we can swim, riding the waves, choosing even to float on our backs at times, trusting the buoyancy of the waves to carry us.

Similarly, we can ride the waves of the breath, accepting that sometimes we will gasp in awe or in horror, sometimes the breath will become ragged with exertion or anxiety, and sometimes the breath will become shallow or stagnant. In each moment, the breath is with us, differing in its texture, tempo, and temperature.

The fluctuations may be subtle or profound. Inhale slowly. Exhale slowly. This breath is exactly the same as the one before, and it is completely different as well.

When we ride the waves of time, of breath, of emotion, of thought, we enter the fluidity of the experience of life. We begin to be able to maintain our center even as we flow.

ॐ Setting an Intention

Each morning when our eyes open, infinite possibilities for the day's rhythm and texture are present. Although many aspects of the day are beyond our control, one thing that *is* in our control is the opportunity to set an intention.

When you first wake up, do you set an intention for the day? The intention may not necessarily be about what you are going to do, but perhaps how you're going to go about it. For instance, instead of setting an intention to work eight hours, your intention might be to stay as calm as possible during those eight hours. At the end of the day, you can check to see how well your intention was met.

Similarly, you can set an intention for your yoga practice as you are driving to class, before you get out of the car, as you are walking in, or even as you are getting on your mat waiting for class to begin. Your intention might simply be to stay fully present throughout class without letting your mind wander away, which is actually not that simple at all. A modified intention might be to notice when your attention wanders and to bring the attention back to the breath. At the end of class or as you are on your way home, you might notice what effect, if any, your intention had on your practice.

You may also wish to dedicate your practice to someone, something, or some place, concept, or ideal that is important to you. In this way, your practice—every breath, every movement, every pose—becomes an offering of light and love.

ॐ Facets

From any angle, the light
strums against the small face
of this moment, its surface
chiseled gently by the breath
washing in and out like tidewater
calmly moving back and forth
seemingly effortlessly like the pulse
keeping us here alive in our skin
while all around us jet streams
of information and misinformation
cloud our skies with threats of fronts
moving in. The moon with its many faces
does not buy into this, the dark jewels
of fear outshone by the wild, sweet glow
of a light that feeds upon night,
leaving bright shadows in its wake.

ॐ Anchoring in the Sea

Have you ever had the chance to be by the sea when a storm is brewing? If so, you may have seen the whitecaps that form as the waves increase exponentially in height and strength. Have you seen the glimmer of sun on water turn suddenly to a heavy gray? The changing nature of the tides and the unpredictable shifts of weather are timeless. Even with Doppler radar, Mother Nature humbles us, keeping us guessing.

Similarly, there are shifting tides and weather patterns in our lives. What can seem like a balmy relaxed day at the beach can become a beach evacuation and a hurricane warning all in an instant. So when these times of uproar come, what or who are your anchors? How do you keep your ship from being swept out to sea? Which yoga pose helps you to find your center? Which yoga pose helps you to feel most grounded, calm, stable, and strong?

ॐ Resistance

D o you sometimes feel too busy to practice yoga? Do you ever decide to do your practice later after you've finished all of your other "stuff" (work, errands, dishes, laundry, phone calls, etc.) and then realize, as you're dropping off to sleep at night, that "later" never came—or it came and you missed it?

With so many things vying for our attention, it's a wonder that yoga is even practiced at all. Even if there is not any external interference and your schedule allows time for a yoga class or a home practice session, there may be internal resistance in the form of feeling too tired, too stiff, too anxious, too distracted, too unworthy to spend the time or money on yourself, or any number of other factors, leading to the idea of practicing yoga being abandoned.

Sometimes rest is best. However, when time for yoga class turns into watching TV or surfing online and eating junk food, then it can be worth it to look a little more closely at what is going on. Is this a one-time anomaly, or is this a pattern of avoiding (intentionally or subconsciously) practice? Sit with this. Perhaps talk about it or write out what you notice. Is it time to begin again or wait a while longer?

ॐ Shipwrecked

I n an instant, our world is rocked. We are underwater, holding our breath, fighting to reach the surface. Or we are treading water, exhausted, the shore too far to reach. Overcome, we drown to our fear, our sorrow, our pain, our anger. And then, there we are, gasping on shore, some impossible moment we cannot escape, splayed open to the all-seeing sun or moon, the ungraspable reach of the unending sky. There is nothing we could say to translate fully the way we have been turned upside down, inside out.

It is our death and re-birth, as the shark's teeth we narrowly missed vanish and we catch our breath, coughing, blinking, our tongues, our minds, split between sea and land, between giving up and getting up, a buoyancy from some deep unseen place offsetting the sinking, and we come to the mat, broken in the most invisible of ways, breathing in the miracle of the shipwreck that has brought us here.

ॐ Upon Waking

Is your waking a gradual rising from the depths of sleep and dream to the surface, drawn by the beckoning of the rising sun, or is it a jolt from the jarring sound of an alarm clock? Do you wake refreshed and ready to embrace the day, or is there a sluggishness, a resistance to getting out of bed? Regardless of your path to waking, there will be a first thought. This thought, washed in the newness of morning, has the potential to shape the entire day. Notice what this thought is. Is there immediately a frantic inventory of the day's tasks? Is there a thought of coffee, food, checking emails/texts, or something else?

The transition from sleep to wake is a prime opportunity to charge the soul with an affirmation, a prayer, a chant, a goal, a scripture, an intention. Just as we learn to pay attention to the charge on the battery of our cell phone or laptop, we can learn to bolster our own battery (mind, body, soul) with an infusion of positive, uplifting thoughts. This practice does not need to be limited to our initial waking but can be integrated into any point in the day when shifting from one experience to another, inviting an awakening of consciousness throughout the day.

In yoga practice, too, we can awaken the cellular intelligence in the body by breathing deeply into each *āsana* (physical posture) while staying as aware of as much of the body as possible, awakening the lungs, the spine, the thighs, the inner and outer edges of the feet, the shoulders, the throat, the crown of the head.

ॐ Mountains, Oceans, and Stars

O ur spiritual practice, our *sādhana*, is taking place right now, right where we are, as we accept the mountains that are before us to climb—in our job, in our relationships, and in our practice. Are we the ant staring up at the peaks, or are we seeing the mountains as anthills as we soar above?

Amidst the oceans of information, oceans of love, and oceans of challenges to swim through right now, whether you are in a city or in a desert or in the woods, flow in your practice like a wave in the sea.

There are, regardless of current challenges, so many constellations of light in the form of people and events shining every day in every direction, counterbalancing the dark, literally and metaphorically. Bring the light into your eyes, into your fingertips, into the very essence of who you are as you move through your practice with ease.

The present—with its mountains and oceans and stars—*is* the present, the gift, even as it opens our eyes, our hearts, our minds.

Be here in this presence with its mountains, oceans, and stars, with the cosmos of beauty and heartache and possibility woven into each and every breath.

ॐ Waiting vs. Being

When you walk into the post office to mail a package and see a long line snaking its way from the counter nearly all the way to the door, how long does it take your frustration to fade? Does it stay with you all the way until you reach the counter as you wait and wait and wait? Or, at some point do you surrender, recognizing that you can't change the situation and that this is a time you can practice Mountain Pose? Or that you can silently pray or practice a *mantra* or an affirmation? Or that you can enjoy observing the facial expressions and body language of the others in this temporary community or even speak with the person next to you? Or that you can simply practice being— being content with where you are, accepting what cannot be changed about the situation?

The world offers us many lines, especially at the airports, when we go to check our bags or go through security. We have the choice to wait in the line or to be in the line. And if we think of our life as a line from start to finish—are we waiting in this line or are we in the line, observing and enjoying as many moments as we can? Are you in this moment now, or are you waiting for the next moment to begin?

ॐ Geology of Breath

From the cliff of bone
to the sea of breath
to the raw pit of fire
just barely beginning to burn
inside a muscle, a thought,
the open space between

From the centrifugal imaginings
spinning out from memories
misplaced, replaced,
not quite erased
to the hidden caves of doubt
collapsing in the shaking
of the earth of the flesh

From the genetic glide
of all things past,
slim fossils imprinted
on the undersides of bones,
to the new cells blossoming
in quiet spaces unseen,
the breath in all seasons
warming the corridor of the spine

ॐ Heart

The enormous elephants in Africa have hearts, the gibbons swinging and leaping high in the trees of North India have hearts, the seals in Ireland that flap their flippers and bark have hearts; even the tiny gnats we may swat away from our face have hearts, and yes, we, too, have hearts—every single one of us—from the prisoners overflowing the jails around the globe to the world's saints to everyone in between.

We have young hearts, old hearts, broken hearts, hearts clogged with plaque, hearts that skip a beat. We have the complexity of the physiological and anatomical heart, we have the energetics of the heart *chakra*, and we have the heart that we can feel, placing our hand on top of the left side of the chest.

Notice your heart's rhythm. As you keep your hand resting on the heart, allow the breath to soften and slow. Feel the communion between your palm and the pumping of the heart. The inhale and exhale come naturally, just as the heart continues beating through our long hours of working and sleeping, when the heart is perhaps the last thing on our mind.

Visualizing the interior of the chambers of your heart, notice where joy, light, and exhilaration are streaming in; notice, too, any areas of heaviness, cloudiness, or dampness. This tremendous vessel of wisdom holds it all.

As the attention stays at the heart, visualize the heart as the sea; observe the sunlight on the ocean waves glimmering as far as the eyes can see. Breathe into this infinite beauty; breathe into love, forgiveness, compassion, and peace. Let these waters wash over the rocky, jagged places that may also reside in the heart. Breathe. Be at home in your heart in the ever-changing presence of now.

ॐ Laughter

Laughter, opening us to joy,
where are you?

Do you breathe with us
as we practice?

In the midst of *āsana*
or meditation will you visit?

You, spirals of delight,
wiser than an hour of study,
alighting on our shoulders,
hips, ankles, the ridges of our spine,

brush us with your light-heartedness,
move like a peacock feather
across the corners of our mouth,
be the joyous light in our heart, our eyes.

ॐ Tears

Have you ever felt tears coming as you practiced yoga, perhaps in the middle of a class? Were you startled because you weren't feeling particularly sad and, in fact, had been in a good mood before the tears inexplicably welled up? Yoga, in its multidimensional capacity to unite the mind, body, and spirit, cleanses subtle, profound, and often buried pathways of emotion. When we open an area of the body, such as the hips, through gentle stretching, we may free blockages in cellular memory that may have been formed years or even decades ago; thus, tears may flow. While it may feel surprising, confusing, frustrating, or even shameful to have this upsurge of emotion, especially if it is in a public place and especially if there doesn't seem to be a logical reason to explain why it's happening, tears can actually be a gift of cleansing or even a form of devotion to the process of healing in the various forms it may take along the journey.

Crying is a natural event, just like yawning or coughing. As with anything in life, balance is vital. If there is an absence of tears in a life or an excess of tears in a life, this may be something to explore further, and just as a river may surge after a storm or a current may be extreme after a dam breaks, variations in the flow of tears within a life may simply be part of a natural flow of cause and effect. If we open our minds to the wisdom of the body, we can free the definition of tears to expand beyond sadness into tears of joy, tears of amazement, tears of laughter, tears of fatigue, and tears of mystery. Tears as sacred messengers invite us to wake up and pay attention to the present moment and its many layers, both seen and unseen.

ॐ Excavation

The trapdoor of the shoulder
leads to the *Well, I couldn't possibly*
part of the soul. It tunnels beneath
the city of unspokenness. A city folded
into itself like a bad dream.
The shoulder, content to hinge
arm to chest, will not mention
any of this. It will deny it
if asked. Instead, it will continue
to protect the hidden world
of the past by reaching forward
and further. Then, in the quiet,
from deep below, a wailing will rise up
in a slight pulsing, a circling soreness.
The cry of a city abandoned.
Waiting. Even Pompeii, buried by lava
and centuries, saw the sun again.
The trapdoor cannot be bolted.
A vein of consciousness, a breath,
it beats in time with time.

ॐ The Undertow

Have you ever stood in the ocean when there was a strong undertow and felt yourself being drawn deeper into the water? There can be a natural healthy undertow in yoga where one practice brings such relaxation or relief or inspiration that we are already looking forward to the next.

However, there can also be an undertow phenomenon that pulls us back into anything other than yoga when we reach points of resistance, mentally, emotionally, or physically.

After all, it can feel awkward and vulnerable to move into the unknown. Even trying to learn how to write the letters of the *Devanāgarī* alphabet, the script used in Sanskrit, can make the mind feel like it is trying to do back flips. With daily practice, though, we can begin writing entire words in *Devanāgarī* like योग (yoga). Similarly, the seemingly endless layers and levels of yoga can serve to fascinate and inspire us, or they can frustrate and overwhelm us as we so choose.

Yoga is a lifelong learning process and if being "good at yoga" means how authentically we feel in each moment of our practice and our life (rather than which poses we can do or how expertly we do them), then we can continue practicing and learning even until the last days of our lives. Even if confined to bed in illness or old age, the oceans of *prāṇāyāma* (breath practices) and meditation are available.

Will you be pulled closer to your practice today or further away?

ॐ Receiving the Teachings

Who are your teachers—past and present? These could be formal teachers from a class or school, mentors, some wisdom coming in from cyberspace, insects or other members of the animal kingdom, plants, children, elders, strangers, family members, life experiences, a piece of music or art, or your very own self.

What have you learned from yourself about yourself? What can you learn from the sky, a tree? Even in the rawest experiences when we are nearly too angry or scared or grief-stricken to breathe, there is a teaching waiting for us as a specially designed gift we can choose to either accept or not.

What do you choose to learn from your breath during your practice today? How closely will you listen to what the muscles and nerves and bones of your body are saying? What about your mind? Can the mind learn from itself? If you were to sit as a student in the school of your heart today, what might you discover?

ॐ Autopilot

One way to move through a yoga class is to listen to the instructions, watch the teacher, watch those students who might be in our line of sight, and try to match what we hear and see (or to simply go into the pose on autopilot). Another way to move through a yoga class is to take in the verbal and visual cues while integrating this with what we are noticing and feeling within our own self. While this may seem like a subtle difference, and to some extent it is, it can make all the difference in the world.

To bring this comparison into sharper focus, consider a specific pose. Let's take Tree Pose, which may be a pose that you have been in hundreds if not thousands of times. One approach would be to move quickly into the pose of standing on one leg while pressing the sole of the other foot into the calf or thigh of the standing leg, concentrating on how well your pose matches what you think you're supposed to be doing. Another approach is to move slowly into the pose, taking note of where the bulk of your weight is balancing on the sole of the foot of the standing leg. See if you can feel the sole of the foot of the bent leg pressing into the standing leg. Is there a kinesthetic conversation where these two meet? Have you contracted your upper body in the process? If you have raised your arms, are your shoulders reaching up towards your ears, or are they relaxed? Where can you feel your breath?

Feeling our way through life can feel like a slower and possibly unnecessary path, especially in a culture that prizes efficiency and quick results. However, there is value in authenticity and innovation, both of which come from a genuine exploration from an original perspective. What is more original than your very own self?

Once we become familiar with the step-by-step process of slowing down, observing, and feeling as we move into a pose, as we stay in a pose, and as we move out from a pose, we can begin to integrate this process into our daily lives as well. Instead of trying to apply a standard template to every situation and conversation, what happens when we begin exploring, noticing someone's tone of voice, facial expression, choice of words, and pauses between words in a conversation? What happens when we immerse ourselves in fully listening to another without concurrently planning what our response is going to be? What becomes possible when we open our heart and mind, moving in and out of each exchange with the awareness of moving into Tree Pose as if for the first time?

ॐ Interwoven

In the center of the ribs,
in small caves, old ones chant,
invoking the grace of heaven
with the geometry of their prayers,
their words, patterned like constellations,
carving small tunnels of light.

In the center of the eyes:
bright stars carrying the news
from galaxies untranslatable
except in the way the reverberation
of a church bell encompasses centuries
sharing the same central sound.

In the center of the palms,
slight etchings of generations
crisscrossing in gentle pathways
not unlike the way one breath
braids briefly with another,
one moment giving birth to the next.

ॐ Coming into Tune

At the beginning of an orchestra's performance, the musicians work to bring their instruments into tune so that the orchestra can function as a healthy organism, doing its *dharma* (life purpose or duty) in bringing concertos, sonatas, and other musical creations to life. Similarly, when the various instruments within us (liver, heart, kidneys, lungs, colon, spleen, eyes, brain) are tuned and working properly, we have a better chance of being in harmony with ourselves and the environment, maximizing our potential to do our life's work as well as to enjoy life's compositions, which we are given the chance to sight-read, either with fear or with faith. *Prāṇāyāma* (breath work), meditation, and *āsana* (physical postures) can help keep our systems toned and tuned.

As you move into your yoga practice, listen for the symphony of each *āsana*. Where is the harmony and dissonance in your Tree Pose, your Downward Dog, your Bridge, your Warrior, your Seated Twist? Watch and feel how your muscles, bones, nerves, and organs work together to create each pose. Notice what is moving more—your mind or your body. Is there synchronicity in the rhythm of body, mind, and soul? Observe the music (or cacophony) that forms in you as the individual *āsanas* come together in different sequences. You may even wish to see how listening to a specific type of music affects the feel and pace of your practice.

ॐ This Is Then, That Was Now

How often do we live in the past, mulling or stewing over conversations that have long since ended, circumstances that no longer exist, and options that passed long ago?

How often do we spin projections of the future based upon our expectations, our needs, our fears, and our hopes?

How often do either of these practices assist us in gaining a sense of peace or in helping us to meet the situations that we are encountering now?

While it is natural, and at times can even be highly beneficial, to look to the past and to look ahead, giving too much energy and time to these practices can rob us of what we can experience and learn right now.

As you enter a yoga pose, do you find yourself thinking about how you have done this pose—better or worse—before? Do you find yourself getting frustrated if the pose is not working the way it usually has in the past? Do you notice yourself fixating on how you have seen someone else do the pose or how you would like to improve upon the pose in the next breath or the next class?

While it can be supportive to have goals for ourselves both on and off the mat, thinking about a goal or brooding over a failure while on the mat tends to put us in the mind, or, at a minimum, it creates a split between the mind and the body, even as we are inside of a practice of unification. The remedy is usually to return to the breath. With repeated encouragement to return to the breath, we begin to enter the present moment more fully and to invite ourselves to receive both its challenges and its gifts.

Find your breath. Where can you feel it? How does it feel? Is it quick or slow? Smooth or jagged? Place one hand on your chest and one hand on your abdomen. Feel the rise and fall of the wave of breath moving within you now.

ॐ New Day

With generosity and grace, this day is born.

This day, not the day that breathed yesterday
or the day that has yet to arrive:
today—alive and awaiting our embrace.

Whether it is dawn or noon or the waning hours of night,
this day breathes in us and we breathe in this day.

What has this day, like a saint, laid before us?
What has this day, like a warrior, placed in our path?

Will we retreat, locking the door and closing the blinds?
Or onto the gradually unfolding path will we step forward?

Into our exquisitely designed hands,
this day keeps arriving,
moment by ever-changing moment
challenging us, welcoming us,

moment by ever-fleeting moment
renewing.

ॐ Chapters of Our Practice

With each breath, each thought, each feeling, each action, we shape the daily-evolving chapters of our life. As we continue practicing yoga, there may be times when we are practicing while recovering from an illness, injury, or deep loss. We may find ourselves practicing in the midst of a new job or relationship.

At some points, a daily practice may occur rather effortlessly, whereas at other times making it to one practice a week may feel like a major accomplishment. Although we might feel inclined to judge ourselves, if we compare what seems like a better chapter of our yoga journey with a weaker one, this will tend to weigh us down, just like comparing our current chapter with another person's chapter.

When we can accept where we are with compassion, this can help us to be fully present in the current stage or season of our life; we can also aim to be fully present in each *āsana*, embracing yoga as a place where we can be in grief, in confusion, in clarity, in peace, in anxiety, in joy, or in any other emotion. Tears spilling onto the mat are not a sign of failure but a sign of a genuine commitment to be present in the practice, regardless of whatever is flowing through.

As you step onto your mat, a page in the current chapter of your life, consider that the stories that came before and the stories that are not yet written pale in comparison to the presence of the breath, the way it is moving through you today in the singular moment of now.

ॐ Language of Light

What is the nature of the words that have been circulating through your mind today? These could be words spoken or unspoken. Are they mostly vibrant light-giving, life-affirming words? Are they dull, murky, heavy words? Are they words as sharp as porcupine quills? Or are they words stirred up like leaves whirling in the wind? Our words, moving swiftly through our being in the form of thoughts circulating like blood through our veins, are a potent presence.

Though our thoughts cannot be seen and are difficult to measure, we can certainly feel their presence, whether they are neutral, bright, or shadowy. Imagine a language of light moving through you, through your veins right now. See it. See the glow of this energy moving throughout your entire body—your head, your throat, your heart, your arms, your core, your legs, right down to your feet.

What does it mean to cultivate a language of light? Does it mean that difficult topics cannot be expressed? No, it simply means choosing to communicate internally and externally at the highest vibration possible. By infusing our thoughts and words with awareness, we can invoke the essence of what it means to communicate holistically with intention, integrity, inspiration, and illumination.

ॐ Not Knowing

The abundance of information that exists in our universe today and the ease of locating data with search engines seem to suggest that answers to all of our questions are available. Can we look online, though, to understand what is expressing through our hip when it moves in a new way in an *āsana*? What book or website can discern the emotion that is emerging from a sequence of poses or from a period of silent meditation? If we determine that the only true source of this knowledge or wisdom resides within the self, what if we cannot answer the questions?

In the way that a hollyhock seed may or may not know the exact colors it will trumpet boldly in the sun one day, we may know and not know. If we know, we may not know *how* we know, and it may be just as important to be comfortable with bursts of intuition arriving from a logic that we don't know how to explain as it is to accept the vast terrain that unfolds when we can admit that we don't know, or perhaps that we know two (or more) things that seem to contradict each other. Maybe you dread and look forward to your yoga practice at the same time. Maybe you are, at the same time, learning to relax more while also becoming more alert, energized, and aware. Maybe the deepest part of the ocean of yourself knows more than reaches the surface. Breath, with its experiential knowledge of every millimeter of the body, may know more than all of the anatomy books combined.

What does the bottom of the foot know? What does the palm know? What is the knowledge of the throat, the spine? Sometimes we may know too much for our own good; sometimes we lack common sense. Returning to the present moment through the wise guide of the breath, how fully can we accept all that we know, as well as all that we do not know without pressing ourselves towards an answer? Waves of possibility abound.

ॐ Of Flexibility and Strength

T he trees that survive decades of storms are usually both strong and flexible. Whether in *Vṛkṣhāsana* (Tree Pose) or any other pose, these two qualities are important in yoga practice. Often, we come to the practice of yoga either with more strength or more flexibility. If we observe others in a yoga class, we can usually see this tendency towards muscular strength, stability, and stamina or towards the ease of flexible movement. While both qualities are necessary, bringing the two qualities into equilibrium will allow us to inhabit our body more fully as well as increase our capacity to enter each *āsana* fully, embodying it—mind, body, and soul.

The resonance of these qualities of strength and flexibility extends outside of *āsana* practice as well. While being flexible (adaptable, amenable, fluid, versatile) can be beneficial up to a point, after a certain point this flexibility can become overly tolerant, capricious, mercurial, fickle, unpredictable, or inconsistent. Similarly, the strength, solidity, robustness, and fortitude that can be a great asset in personal and business relationships can become forcefulness or insistence when taken to an extreme.

As we come into balance through a dedicated practice, we can learn to adapt and flow even as we remain strong, and we can learn to become stronger even as we remain flexible. Thinking back to when you first began to practice yoga, what is one pose that you feel stronger in now? In which pose do you feel more flexible? While we can't always feel our strength or flexibility improving day to day, it can become noticeable when we pause and reflect on our earlier self versus our current self—the strength of our convictions, the flexibility and fluidity of our movement—both on and off the mat.

ॐ Balancing Act

Have you tried reciting the alphabet backwards while standing on one leg? Coordinating two things at once is not always as easy as it seems. For instance, sometimes we are so focused on maintaining our balance in a pose that we lose track of our alignment, or we're so focused on alignment that we tighten and contract. Similarly, if we focus our attention on others' needs excessively, we can lose sight of our own. Conversely, if we focus too much on our own self, we can forget the needs and feelings of others. It is a balancing act both on and off the mat. Even if we are not in a balancing pose, we are finding the balance between placing our attention on the mind and on the body.

At some point along the way, we can begin to focus externally while simultaneously focusing internally. As we listen to another, we, at the same time, can listen to ourselves, noting our reactions, our judgments, and our observations. As we look at another person, we can concurrently look closely at ourselves, recognizing our shared humanity. As we balance the exhale of our outward-moving energy with the inhale of inward-moving energy, we can begin to create a balanced whole.

Take a moment now and count the length of your in-breath; count the length of your out-breath. What is the capacity for expansion for what you take in as well as what you release?

ॐ Feet

Our feet, the brave loyal ones connecting us to the ground, are unsung heroes. We may glance at them as we slip on shoes or put on socks, but often that is the extent of the attention they receive from us, unless we stub our big toe, develop a blister on the heel, or step on something sharp. Yet, without our feet, where would we be? Daily, moment by moment, our feet carry us, making it possible for us to start and stop, to tend to the business of our days.

Our feet, delivering us again and again to the present moment, often do so without receiving our appreciation. Still, they carry on, humble and devoted.

To observe a map of the bottom of the foot that shows which points of the foot relate to specific internal organs and specific parts of the body is to be awed by the careful and loving design of our bodies, right down to the soles of our feet.

With one sole of the foot on the ground and one sole of the foot on the calf or thigh, we balance in *Vṛkṣhāsana* (Tree Pose). In *Dhanurāsana* (Bow Pose), our soles lift to the sky. In *Trikoṇāsana* (Triangle Pose) and *Vīrabhadrāsana II* (Warrior 2 Pose), we place our feet wide apart, the quiet choreography of the foot placements in a series of *āsanas* leaving invisible impressions on the ground. *Baddha Koṇāsana* (Bound Angle) brings the soles of our feet together as if they are two palms pressed together in prayer, or opening as the covers of the book we are writing with every step of our lives.

Look down at your feet. Move your feet. Touch your feet. Remember how tiny your feet once were. Bring to mind the many miles these feet have crossed, the ground, the sand, the gravel, the concrete, the mud, the floors made of wood, marble, adobe, or linoleum they have walked upon. Thank your ten toes for leading the way, as they do, as they have, as they will, step after step after step.

ॐ Hands

S it in a comfortable cross-legged position.

Connect with your breath. Follow its flow in and out.

Bring your palms together at your heart. Breathe.

Bring your hands, palms up, so that they are resting on your lap.

Observe your palms. Notice the unique patterns of lines woven into them.

Notice each one of your fingers, starting with the thumb and moving to the little finger.

Notice similarities and differences in the two hands. Moving your palms close to your face, look at the color of your hands, their textures.

Turn your hands over, and again, observe. Are the nails smooth, shiny, ridged, long, short?

Take one hand and move it over the other hand, noticing what you feel.

Is the hand warm or cool? Rough or smooth? Moist or dry? Are there any places of stiffness or pain?

Press your right thumb into the center of the left palm, applying gentle pressure. Then, take the left thumb and press it into the right palm.

As you close your eyes, think about all of the things your hands have touched today. Bring to mind all of the actions your hands have performed for you—holding items such as your hairbrush, toothbrush, spoon, and steering wheel, unlocking the door, opening the door, locking the door, helping you to get dressed, typing texts and emails, hugging someone you love, and the list goes on. Thank your hands, bringing them back to your lap.

As you move through your practice, notice what your hands do. Feel the palms press into the ground in Downward Dog; feel the hands press together at the heart or reach up to the sky in Tree Pose; feel the fingertips extend to opposite sides of the room in Warrior 2; feel the backs of the hands rest against the floor in *Shavāsana*.

For now, rub the palms together, generating warmth, and then place them gently over your eyes. Then, gradually moving the hands away, open your eyes, gazing into your palms. As you return to the light of day, place your palms together at your heart. *Namaste.*

ॐ *Honoring the Light*

What does your life salute? In many parts of the world, those in the military pause and raise the right hand to the forehead as an acknowledgement of respect when encountering a military officer. Similarly, there are many ways we salute on a daily basis, such as giving our time and attention to what we consider important. We may salute begrudgingly or whole-heartedly, but without a doubt, our lives are characterized by where we spend our time and what we are doing with that time.

What do you honor in your practice of yoga? Do you focus more on the body, breath, mind, or spirit? The word "*namaskāra*," meaning "salutations," appears in the names of the yoga sequences *Sūrya Namaskāra* (Sun Salutations) and *Chandra Namaskāra* (Moon Salutations). Bringing a *Namaskāra* sequence into your morning practice, perhaps the warmth of *sūrya* to offset the cold of winter, or the cooling nature of *chandra* to offset the heat of summer, is a way to express gratitude for the sources of light in our lives.

Quite literally, the bright heat of the sun allows daylight to come, helping us to see and helping plants to grow. The cool luminosity of the moon shines through the darkest of nights, and the transformation of its shape reminds us of the changing nature, the impermanence of our lives.

The sources of light in our life are abundant. Light may come in an inspiration, a song, a poem, a photograph, a painting, a prayer, a dream. Our days and nights contain such rich sources of light, whether they are hidden or obvious. By turning our attention to them, we salute them inwardly, silently, reminding ourselves of our priorities, gratitude, and respect. We can also choose to outwardly salute, verbally or in writing, someone whose efforts bring light to the world.

Pressing our palms together at the heart, either literally or metaphorically, we honor the light in ourselves and in our friends, colleagues, neighbors, loved ones, and strangers, for even in the darkest of nights, there are, however dimly shining, remarkably luminous stars.

ॐ Dialogue Within

As the vessel of our body moves through a series of poses in a yoga class or in a practice at home, it is traveling, at times, through uncharted waters. In the end, we are all in the same boat. Sometimes the weather—internally or externally—is clear and all goes well. Other times, however, an unseen iceberg is encountered or stirred-up waters can begin knocking us off course.

A mutiny can break out inside with thoughts proclaiming that a pose is too difficult, that we don't have the strength or flexibility to do it or stay in it; the internal voices can then begin criticizing the body's abilities or the teacher's expectations or any other factor that may be chosen to blame. All this inner commentary and commotion does, in the end, is further rock the boat, threatening to send the crew—the many facets of our awareness—overboard. Meanwhile, if we check to see who or what is at the helm (Is it fear? Is it worry? Is it poor self-esteem?), we can often realize and regain our composure.

In regaining our composure, our balance begins to steady. We see that we do not have to judge ourselves so harshly after all. If we are moving intentionally through our practice with integrity, we can, once we hear the inner mutiny begin, soften our experience and soften our expression so that, even when we feel something capsizing, we can stay with the breath, keeping us from sinking or jumping ship. Staying in the center of the practice, whatever it is bringing, we gain, eventually, stamina, endurance, resilience, and calm.

As you move through your practice today, both on and off the mat, notice what type of commentary is taking place inside. Listen closely. Is it ruled by logic, intuition, love, fear, or something else? Breathe deeply, remembering who you are, tapping into the wellspring of infinite wisdom and grace within.

ॐ Internal Landscape

Our bodies are our most familiar territory, and yet they can, at times, feel like foreign lands. There are mysteries in our nerves, muscles, and bones that we may never understand. Our mind inhabits a cosmos unto itself, and our heart, lungs, liver, spleen, pancreas, thyroid, and cerebellum are sometimes like planets spinning in their own orbits. A cartographer would be hard-pressed to chart every line and crevice in our miraculous skin. A geographer could try to track and explain the river of every vein, artery, and capillary and to understand the subtle tectonics of every cell. And yet, the synergy of the systems of our body—respiratory, urinary, reproductive, digestive, neuromuscular, immunological, and more—involves the integration of entire continents, with millions of activities happening at the micro-level on a moment-by-moment basis. Truly, we are scientific wonders and works of art.

In terrain as vast and complex as our bodies, it is not surprising that the years can bury and obscure much, just as the shifting sands and weather patterns of our environment can hide things from our sight. We may be in the midst of a familiar pose and suddenly find an unexpected emotion, memory, or idea appearing. It could be a sensation of fear, anger, worry, joy, peace, or something else. Where did it come from? Why and how is it arising from the particular configuration of the body and breath at that moment? While we may or may not see or feel a logical connection, the experience itself is real, and to simply feel it and acknowledge it is part of a valuable excavation of Self.

Just as there can be an excavation where anthropologists and archaeologists go out on an expedition with a mission, there can be a more spontaneous experience of layers when a shard of pottery or the skeleton of a winged dinosaur or the architecture of an ancient civilization is uncovered unexpectedly. And just as the earth is a record of prior events and time, the body, too, stores an accumulation of experiences, not just in the brain but in the entire cellular structure of the body as well as at the subtle level of the emotions.

Āsana (yoga poses), *prāṇāyāma* (breath practices), *dhāraṇā* (concentration), and *dhyāna* (meditation) are just some of the many paths of purification that can cleanse and clear what may have accumulated in our bodies over time. As we open to the process of exploration, the excavation naturally occurs.

Minute Meditations

ॐ   Heart Song

May your heart know peace
May your heart know joy
May your heart receive
May your heart give
Place your hand at your heart
and feel the waves of love shining within

ॐ Morning Song

May the day ahead of you unfold beautifully,
every molecule of yesterday gracefully releasing
May your mind and heart open
like a morning glory to the sun
May you, washed clean by the moon
and the breath deep in your lungs, begin anew

ॐ   Evening Song

May you be released from the events
of the day replaying in your mind
May your bones, muscles, and nerves
welcome the relaxation of rest
May you find an oasis of quiet
and take refuge there,
nourishing the space
where the essence of your soul resides

ॐ Moment Song

In this moment, may you be at peace
What has come before has already passed
What is yet to be has not yet arrived
Enter fully into this breath, this moment,
tasting it, hearing it, feeling it, seeing it,
knowing it, accepting it, breathing it,
cherishing this singular ephemeral experience
receding already into the cosmic sea

ॐ Illusion

W hat is real and what is not? What is fake and what is true? Is something synthetic or organic? Does either make it more or less real? Is something authentic just because it has been labeled as such? Is something real or true just because it is online or in print? With the ever-increasing challenges of recognizing and understanding the veracity of what is tangible, it is no wonder that we find challenge in discerning what is real and what is not within the intangible realms of our mind and heart.

Illusion has been a deceptive force since ancient times when a rope may have been mistaken to be a snake, and yet illusion is also a teaching tool, a possibility for growth. Getting to the point where we might be able to consider, on a regular basis, whether a thought or a belief may be an illusion presenting itself convincingly as truth is significant; however, as with anything, finding a balanced stance is key. If we allow uncertainty to move into excess, we can become hypervigilant or even paranoid. A certain amount of skepticism can be healthy, but just as we would likely not pour an entire salt shaker of salt on our food, we can benefit from not saturating our minds with doubt.

In time, with the practice of awareness, our sense of what is accurate and authentic tends to develop and become more reliable. However, the very nature of illusion is that it is very clever, and even the brightest, most experienced yogis can fall prey to its influence.

Self-study (*svādhyāya*) can help us to investigate which patterns in our thinking may be affected by illusory influences. It can also be helpful to talk with someone who has an objective point of view so that we can hear the way our thoughts sound when spoken aloud, and so that we can receive an honest response and a wider perspective.

As we move into our practice, the breath can be our guide as well. As we breathe more deeply into a pose or a part of the body, the sensation can change. Which sensation is real? Which is illusion? Could they all be real? Could they all be illusion? Let go of trying to solve the puzzle. Return to the breath. If your breath were not real, would you be here?

ॐ Quieting the Waves of the Mind

The use of the word "mindful" has increased exponentially. The increased usage of this word suggests that what was once a natural way of being—aware, conscious, sensible, alert, wise, cognizant—is something that we need to be reminded of now and even coached or encouraged to incorporate into our lives. This is not surprising given the increased pace of life, the influx of electronics, and the shift to 24-hour global connectivity.

If the mind is full, perhaps even to overflowing, what does it take to become mindful? Sometimes a downsizing of our schedule is needed, but often it is simply through prioritizing our practice that a shift into a more balanced lifestyle can occur. This prioritizing can take the form of building ten minutes of meditation into the daily schedule, perhaps first thing in the morning before being swept away by the day. It can also come in the form of choosing to participate in a yoga class or in another experience that is calming and quiet.

More can be more, and more can be less. Through careful discernment, we can consider each day what the wisest choices will be. Sometimes it is best to exert effort to push forward while sometimes it is best to let go and rest. Our innate wisdom of the body-mind-soul will let us know as we learn to tune into it on an ongoing basis. Just as we sometimes benefit from holding a pose longer than we thought we could, sometimes the benefit is in coming out of a pose, taking an alternative pose or counterpose, or simply resting.

Whether the meter of the mind registers full or empty or somewhere in between, as inner awareness grows, the waves of the mind can begin to become quiet and calm.

ॐ Continuity

T hink for a moment about your journey here to the mat. Whether you were walking, bicycling, driving, riding in a bus or car, what was your state of mind? Were you in silence, listening to music, or perhaps talking on the phone? Were you worried that you were running late? Were you looking forward to arriving? Did you feel off-kilter or balanced and calm?

Similarly, what happens when we move out of our yoga practice and into the world? If we exit class, get into the car, and begin driving only to honk the horn in frustration at another driver, how well has the practice been integrated into our overall life? If we stop on the way home to buy groceries and become very impatient waiting in line, how well are we digesting the fruits of the practice in moments like this when the person on the mat may not seem to match the person moving about in the world?

Integration is a process that does not happen overnight, so we do not need to despair or give up when we notice parts of our lives that seem to be out of alignment. In some cases, a strong dose of compassion is indicated, and in other cases, a strong dose of discipline (*tapas*) may be required. Each situation is different; each person is different, and each of us is different in each unfolding moment.

The next time you come to the mat, notice how you move into your practice, through your practice, and out of your practice into the rest of your life, noticing where your life and practice are in alignment and where the two diverge.

ॐ The Current, the River, and the Rain

The riverwaters gleam
a glistening black, the recent rainwaters
quivering the current. It is night
and there is nowhere to go
but everywhere. The spilling of one thread
into the next.
 And this flow
does not stop does not stop does not stop.
It opens into the wingspan of morning
coasting in over the night's sprawl,
over the first sleep, second sleep,
last sleep.
 The river of breath
spilling over the crests and banks
of the bones, slipping in and out
of the corridors of the lungs,
sending its currents rippling into the farthest reaches
of toe tips and palms,
 the curl and curve
of all that gives and all that gives way,
the edges letting go into something softer,
sweeter, the mirage of goodbye breaking
apart,
 the weight of a construction crane
reduced to a bright yellow leaf floating
on the Gihon River which is Powell River
and the Potomac and the Rio Grande and every river
brushing the earth with smooth, sure strokes
shaping the tides of live and the tides of die
that speak each time we breathe.

ॐ Washing Clean

We have entire rooms devoted to washing—laundry rooms with washing machines to clean our clothes and elaborate showers and bathtubs for washing the body. Where is the room dedicated to washing the mind, the heart? If there is not space for a meditation room, is there an area dedicated to meditating, *prāṇāyāma*, chanting, *āsana*, prayers, or other spiritual practices?

How about your mat? With a shift of attention, the yoga mat can become a space of respite, sanctuary, and awareness.

When was the last time you cleaned your mat? By washing our mat lovingly, we pay respect by removing the vestiges of dust as well as our sweat and tears; we also pay respect to what the mat symbolizes, which is likely something different to each person. Maybe your *āsana* practice is about getting in shape or staying in shape. Maybe it's about keeping stiff muscles and joints at bay. Maybe it's about stress management, or maybe it's part of a path towards spiritual liberation.

How often to clean a yoga mat will vary from person to person. Similarly, how often we cleanse our heart and mind will likely vary. There can be a daily meditation practice, or there may be a simple one-minute pause upon waking and before going to sleep. In that pause in the morning you may wish to make an intention for your day. At night, the pause can give space to review the day, both its challenges and its gifts. Even these short, simple pauses can begin to cleanse the heart and mind.

If we don't clean our office and living space a little bit each day, things can rather quickly get out of hand, resulting in an overwhelming mess. The same holds true for the rooms and passageways of our heart and mind.

ॐ The Journey

I n this life, we are traveling pathways daily, whether the path is from the bedroom to the kitchen, from one part of the city or country to another, or even crisscrossing the international skies.

Often, we may commute by car. What happens when the road you are traveling narrows to one lane as you come upon a construction zone? The driving speed limit has been cut in half with "Fines Doubled" signs posted in the area. Do your thoughts speed up or slow down? Perhaps it is a school zone instead of a construction zone. Is your reaction the same? As your vehicle slows to a crawl, your mind is given a chance to slow down as well. Does it?

Perhaps it is not a slow-down in a construction or school zone that you experience but the complete standstill of a traffic jam. There is a sea of red taillights as far as you can see. Do you begin to fume in frustration? An unexpected delay can be disconcerting, whether the delay is on a tarmac or in a terminal or on a freeway; however, once the initial upset has passed, we are free to choose to feel separate and adrift, or connected with those who are also caught in the unexpected situation.

Similarly, in yoga class, observing the mind can lead to feeling frustrated and overwhelmed with six lanes of speeding thoughts zooming past at 90 mph. Consider, however, that even in the peaceful quiet, those around you may also have similarly chaotic minds. See if you can slow this mental traffic in your own mind—as if a construction zone or a traffic jam has appeared. Connect with your breath. Staying present with each full inhale and exhale, feel the internal traffic begin to ease.

ॐ Staying

I n this world of infinite diversions, sometimes the most challenging thing can be simply to stay silent and to stay still—especially when we feel something difficult or even just unfamiliar arising within. For instance, if there is a wave of what feels like it could be grief or insecurity or anger, there can be a tendency to reach for the phone to text or surf the internet, to reach for the TV remote, to reach for some potato chips or cookies, or to reach for any number of other things that may, at least for the time being, allow us some distance from what the mind or heart may feel is unbearable or even just uncomfortable.

Distraction is often a natural instinct to try to protect ourselves from what we don't wish to feel or see, and the distraction can even be something seen as otherwise healthy, like focusing on work or exercise. When we can begin to move away from judging ourselves for feeling like we cannot handle any more stress, we can begin to notice when we are pulling away from ourselves and reaching for something to block a discomfort in our mind or heart.

Yoga class may be the only time we actually slow down and stay within a quiet environment for an extended period of time. Do you ever find to-do lists, grocery lists, plans for the weekend, or memories of last year zipping through your mind as you practice? This is not unusual, especially in early stages of practice, as the habitual patterns of the mind can be fairly deeply ingrained and may tend to be quite stubborn. Keep in mind that each of us will experience the practice of yoga and even each individual class differently—physically, mentally, and emotionally. A class that may be invigorating to someone else may be exhausting to you; a class that might be relaxing and restorative to you might not be stimulating enough for someone else.

Keep in mind, too, that it may take weeks or months to notice how your practice of yoga is shaping the way you eat, move, sleep, and feel. Are you willing to stay with the practice? Even after years of practice, there may be rough patches, whether from a physical ailment, a surge of doubt or lethargy, or turning the attention to other activities. Are you willing to stay, even when it's easier to look away, walk away, or run away from something within?

If our practice of yoga is not confined to the mat, our ability to stay in relationship with life with its array of challenging people and circumstances may expand. Rather than ignoring or avoiding what feels too difficult, we can pay attention to our breath at those moments and see what else emerges. When we can yoke the light of paying attention with the undercurrents of what makes us squirm or cringe or react in some other way, we are truly practicing yoga.

ॐ One Day at a Time

Transformation, especially on the spiritual path, can sometimes seem abstract, elusive, beyond our reach, and yet when we can give our attention to just one step in the journey rather than trying to travel this entire distance instantaneously, we can make steady progress. Dedicating each day to a specific focus is one approach:

- Monday—Meditation/Mat: Take time to stretch and strengthen the body through yoga *āsana* (or another form of exercise that integrates body, mind, and breath). Take five minutes (or more) to practice meditation.

- Tuesday—*Tapas* (self-discipline): Challenge yourself today to work more effectively and efficiently in your vocation or avocation—or in your yoga practice.

- Wednesday—Wait/Watch: Today, pause for a moment (or two) before responding to a situation, feeling, or thought. Watch. Notice what happens—inside and around you.

- Thursday—Thankfulness: Choose to feel appreciation today. Try pausing each hour (or after each *āsana*) to notice what you are grateful for, no matter how small it is.

- Friday—Food: Pay attention today to what you eat, when you eat it, why you eat it, how you eat, and how you feel after your meal is complete.

- Saturday—Simplify: Do you try to pack too much into your weekend or week? Reduce the load. Simplify. Breathe.

- Sunday—Surrender: Are you carrying the weight of the world on your shoulders? Do you try to carry the weight of someone else, too? Let go. Allow yourself to receive support.

ॐ Ceremony: Honoring Each Moment

When you come into yoga class, how does your mat get onto the floor? Do you have any specific recollection of dropping or placing it on the ground, or any particular memory of unrolling it? Were you talking with someone else as you put the mat down? Was there an internal dialogue taking place? While there is not a specific way to set up a yoga mat, when we bring our attention to our actions, we move from a dispersed energy to a focused one, aligning ourselves with now. When we can give a few moments of attention to setting our yoga mat down, it can become a sacred act in which the yoga mat transforms from a rectangle of material to a space of sanctity for the practice. The point is not to create an elaborate ritual but to see what happens when the act is imbued with intention, or even simply with some awareness.

This approach can be applied to each facet of our life. When we approach each *āsana* with reverence, it is less likely that we will do the pose mechanically out of habit. Similarly, if we bring our attention to the details of ordinary processes such as dressing, eating, and driving, we can begin to move out of autopilot and into the present moment. It's not about adding any time to these processes; rather, it is about infusing them with awareness. Each time we sync the actions of our body with our breath and with the movement—or stillness—of our mind, we create alignment. If you've ever been adjusted while in Triangle (*Trikoṇāsana*), or Downward Dog (*Adho Mukha Shvānāsana*), you know how easy it is to be out of alignment—literally—without realizing it.

As we center ourselves in the present, whether we are coughing, chopping broccoli, paying bills, brushing our teeth, or something else, we come into alignment with time and space. Continuing this practice on a regular basis can allow other facets in the prism of life to come into closer alignment, such as alignment with our goals, responsibilities, loved ones, and the environment. Trying to force this alignment will only cause torquing, resistance, or undue tightening; therefore, start small. Choose just one action today to perform with your complete attention. It can be as simple as putting on or taking off your shoes or placing your feet onto your mat with awareness. When we honor each moment, no matter how mundane or seemingly inconsequential, life takes on the sacred beauty of ceremony.

ॐ *Mantra*

To chant in the beautiful ancient language of Sanskrit or to listen to Sanskrit being chanted can be a healing experience. Even to repeat the single syllables of *bīja* (seed) sounds associated with each of the *chakras* can be transformational. There are recordings by Vyaas Houston and others that can assist in this process.

In addition to delving into the vast oceans of Sanskrit, the words and phrases that we repeat in our thoughts and in our mouths tend to shape the vibration of our lives. If you're not sure which words you tend to repeat, ask those who know you well. Clearly "Anything is possible!" is going to have a different effect than "You just can't win" on both the speaker and listeners, especially when the phrase is repeated on a daily basis.

Some of what we say is simply habit—perhaps something we've heard others say that we're echoing without fully realizing it. However, when we speak with intention, we can begin to clear out words and phrases that don't seem to correlate with what we wish our lives to represent. This can take some time, though, so it can help to have humor, smiling or laughing, rather than putting yourself down, when you hear yourself say the same thing—again. You can also experiment with bringing an uplifting word or phrase to mind on a regular basis—once an hour or even once every fifteen minutes. You might also try introducing a new word into your speech each day.

Words have potency, not just in their meanings but also in the energy of their sound. Paying attention to how you feel when you say—or even just think—certain words can guide you to an awareness of sound— and the language that nurtures, empowers, depletes, aggravates, or compromises. Notice how your tongue moves in your mouth and across your palate as you speak. If we approach our speech and our thoughts as *āsanas*, we can begin to communicate more clearly and cleanly, moving into each expression with union of body (mouth/tongue), mind, and spirit. By slowing ourselves down through awareness, we can purify our minds and our words, just as we tone and cleanse the body through *āsana*.

Sometimes we communicate quite a bit without even saying a word. What do your body movements communicate through the silence of your *āsana* practice? What do your facial expressions convey? What does your posture or body language say throughout the day? Translate the non-verbal language of your life to see what it is saying.

Will your life be a *mantra* for love? What kind of resonance will the actions and words of your life create? With both our words and our silence we shape and reflect the world, one breath, one moment, one syllable at a time.

ॐ Infusion of Light

S andalwood, rose, frankincense, amber, jasmine, myrrh. The fragrant scent of a single stick of incense burning can transform the entire atmosphere of a room. If the sunlight is coming in a window near the incense at just the right angle, the beautiful swirling pattern can be seen as it permeates, infusing the air with its aroma.

If you think of your mind as a stick of incense, what is it infusing—into your being and into the environment around you? Is your mind calm? Anxious? In flux? Is it optimistic, considering the best possible outcomes? Is it fixated on doom and gloom? Just as adding the scent of incense will instantly alter the atmosphere, shifting your intention and attention can transform the signals your mind emits.

Try it. What is something you are worried about right now? Bring to mind the best possible outcome, seeing it, hearing it, feeling it, touching it until it seems real.

Then, bring to mind something that saddens you and just observe that grief or hurt, accepting it without trying to change or fix it. Hold the pain as fully, as compassionately, as lovingly as you can. Feel it begin to soften.

As you move into your practice today, what will you infuse into each *āsana*? What will your attitude, your mindset, your intention transmit to your own individual practice and to the room where you are practicing?

May we infuse the wisdom of our practice into the moments of our lives!

ॐ Limitations and Possibilities

Life is an experience of limitations and possibilities. Quite literally, our life is confined to a limit of a certain number of years, which translates into a certain number of moments or breaths. And yet a single breath can feel so expansive.

Similarly, our yoga practice may be limited by the amount of time we can devote to it as well as our energy levels and physical capacities. Even if we are not dealing with a weak ankle or a stiff hip or a sore back, we often have limitations in our minds regarding which poses we can't do or even how long we might be able to hold a pose. And while it's certainly important not to overexert or strain during practice, it's equally important to challenge our comfort zones so that growth can occur. The guidance of an experienced and wise teacher can be especially helpful here. Bringing discipline, or *tapas*, to the practice, can allow deeper levels to emerge.

We can also free ourselves from any fear or frustration associated with what we may perceive to be our limitations by embracing them as qualities that make us unique and as opportunities to exercise compassion, as well as opportunities to grow and change.

Within the current limitations you perceive in yourself right now, what is possible for you today in your practice and in your life? The only real way to find out is to begin.

DIVING DEEPER
Reflections on Yoga

Diving Deeper

Yoga is more than what meets the eye. It is more than the physical postures being practiced in studios, gyms, churches, ashrams, corporate buildings, schools, community organizations, parks, and homes. It is more than the props of blankets, blocks, bolsters, and straps. Yoga is an eight-limbed system of great depth. Even though we do not need to know about the eight limbs or five *kleshas* or seven *chakras* in order to stand in *Vṛkṣhāsana* (Tree Pose), exploring these depths is a way to deepen our practice. The meditations that follow are a way to dip your toes into these ancient waters that are still very much alive today.

Eight Divine Branches

In Patañjali's *Yoga Sūtras*, he states in Sūtra 2.29 that *yama, niyama, āsana, prāṇāyāma, pratyāhāra, dhāraṇā, dhyāna*, and *samādhi* are the eight limbs of yoga.

Yama

Ancient guidelines like the *yamas* may not be trending in social media, and yet these guides, ancient as they are, have great significance, even in the modern world. *Yamas* are guidelines for living. To try to follow even one of the *yamas* 100 percent of the time can be more challenging than performing one *āsana*. *Yamas* comprise the first limb of yoga; therefore, they are the foundation. What if all those who go to the many yoga studios across the world were to first master, or at least regularly practice, the first limb of yoga before embarking upon the physical postures (*āsana*)? How might our world transform if all those who practice yoga were to devote themselves regularly to even just one *yama*? We can begin by pausing to remember the five *yamas*, inviting one or more to enter into our daily consciousness.

The *yamas* are:

ahiṃsā

satya

asteya

brahmacharya

aparigraha.

Keeping a list of the *yamas* (and *niyamas*) in the area where you meditate (or any place where you are likely to see it) can be an easy way to remind the mind to be kind, to be gentle, to be fair.

ॐ Practicing Peace: *Ahiṃsā*

A*hiṃsā* is the practice of non-violence. Nearly every day in the news we see or hear about violent acts of vandalism, murder, terrorism, and other difficult-to-digest situations at the local, national, and international level, yet there are also many internal forms of violence that exist. Within the realm of violence-to-self, for example, there is self-degradation, when judgmental or negative comments appear in the internal dialogue.

Take a scan for a moment through the past day, or even the past hour, and bring to mind any less-than-favorable thoughts you've had about yourself. Assess them for accuracy, for fairness, for mercy, for compassion. Sometimes a negative line of thinking becomes so frequent, so common, so familiar that it blends in and becomes part of the norm, so much that it fails to be detected as foreign or harmful.

Violence also can emerge in the form of criticism of others. This may be outward, such as in verbal complaints or criticism, even escalating to angry shouting and name-calling. It can also be a silent judgment, intentional ignoring, or refusal to reply to correspondence or calls. Sometimes, however, there can be reasons for healthy separation; this is an area that requires genuine discernment.

Clearly, though, there can be negativity at the vibrational level. Body language and facial expression can transmit quite a bit. Picture a person who is glowering, for instance. The power of such non-verbal communication is real. Just as many believe that the positive energy of prayer can have healing effects, even from great distances, it seems that the corollary also holds true: negative thoughts and words can have damaging effects. In contrast to the very obvious forms of violence that can land a person in prison for life, there are subtle acts of violence that can sneak into the consciousness and wreak havoc before the invasion has even been noticed.

As you move through your day, paying attention to the language and images within your internal and external environment, notice any harshness, applying the awareness of *ahiṃsā* to it like gentle but potent salve passed down through many generations.

ॐ In This World (*Ahiṃsā*)

In this world
where violence shakes through,
earthquaking us, right down to our core,

in this world
where we wage war
against our own self,

let us, with eyes open
to the devastation,
choose peace

let us, with hearts open
to the raw sour pain,
choose grace

with hands open,
let us embrace the despair
without becoming despair

While feeling the darkness
of an entire night sky,
feel the light of the moon
glowing within

ॐ Sacred Syllables: *Satya*

atya means "truth." What does it mean to live in truth? First, there is the courageous work of being with what is presently appearing within—even if, and especially if, it's something unpleasant, such as grief, fear, resentment, judgment, anger, or jealousy. This takes great honesty; it is so much easier to look away, to use distractions—food, work, texting, TV, etc.—to pull away from what brings discomfort. Breathe. What you are feeling—whether it is joy, excitement, depression, frustration, or something else is *part* of you—it is not *you*.

The more closely aligned we are with truth internally, the better able we are to communicate with others from a place of truth. This may mean softening into a vulnerability that gives uncertainty permission to speak. It may mean taking the initiative to bring up a topic or start a conversation. Looking into the eyes of your friend or a stranger and seeing yourself in him or her—since we are, after all, more alike than different—is usually a good place to start. When we communicate from a place rooted in the heart, truth has a chance to flower.

What is the truth of this moment for you? Allow this truth to speak from the depths of your being—your cells, your bones, your muscles, your nervous system, your heart, your mind. Allow it to express itself fully, freely, without any editing. Can you allow space within for this truth to have a home?

What space can you offer within your mind and heart for the truths of others, as complicated as they may be? Often the truth of someone's life may surprise us; however, when we offer sincere listening—without preconceptions—we invite the authenticity of life to move closer, challenging our assumptions and revealing the beautiful complexity of creation.

ॐ Rooting into Truth (*Satya*)

In the midst of the antithesis
of honesty, with integrity crumbling
all around, with false information
flying like an epidemic of disease-carrying mosquitoes
thirsty for blood, stay true. Let your mind and mouth
house only what is rooted in truth.

Weed out everything else.
Be discerning. Some poisonous weeds
may appear to be flowers.

Consider your gestures, your actions,
all of your expressions. What do they say?

Are you eclipsing your own authenticity?

Breathe into the truth of who you are.

Place each word on your tongue
with the care you would take
with choosing a tattoo for your face.

ॐ Integrity: *Asteya*

A*steya* is the *yama* that deals with non-stealing. If you've never been charged with grand larceny or shoplifting, does this mean that you are practicing *asteya*? Maybe, maybe not. There are subtler forms of *asteya* that demand an integrity that can be uncomfortable.

For instance, we can steal from ourselves. We can steal opportunities from ourselves, for example, through negative self-talk and choosing not to engage in a possibility, whether it is a job, a relationship, or something else. Additionally, we can steal our own well-being through poor choices of food intake, sleep patterns, and other habits that don't serve our highest good.

What is one choice you have made within the last week that diminished rather than supported your own sense of health, ease, or comfort in this world?

Asteya can also take the form of stealing from the self by not opening ourselves to receive what is being offered by the universe. It may be a kindness or it may be an offer of practical support; the forms are endless. However, if the heart closes through pride or even uncertainty, beautiful experiences can be missed, and stagnation in the flow of energy can build.

The next time someone offers you an unexpected kindness, whether a compliment or something more tangible, see what might happen if you opened yourself to the possibility of receiving it.

Stealing from the self can also take the form of spending time or money on things that don't ultimately support our highest good. For instance, what is the nature of your bank account? Does the direction of your finances reflect your highest values? Similarly, what happens with your 24 hours each day? Are there any activities that are depleting your energy or that are out of alignment with your goals?

In another permutation of *asteya*, we can steal from others by hoarding our energy and talents, withholding them from the world. Certainly, there are finite hours in the day, and if you are a person of many talents, it may not be possible to contribute all of them; however, there are times when we have plenty of capacity to give and do not. This steals from us the experience of sharing and steals from others the experience of receiving.

This, of course, is a delicate line and is something to assess and process individually, for there is also the possibility of stealing from the self by giving too much and not leaving enough time to simply be.

Breathe. Breathe into your true self that intuitively knows the ideal balance of how much to give and how much to receive. Make an intention not to steal from yourself or from others, even at the subtlest levels, and see what changes begin to emerge.

ॐ Can You Steal the Ocean? (*Asteya*)

Move through this life lightly
taking only what you need.

There is enough.
A vast ocean of time,
of energy, of love exists.

If there is one green shoe
sitting alone in the sand, leave it there.
It may be someone's landmark
or abstract sculpture. The one who forgot it
may be on the way back to retrieve it.

Everything is someone's, and, in the end, nothing
is ours. Me, my, mine. You, yours, theirs.
Remove the pronouns. Remove the possession.

Accepting the temporary ownership
of things in this life, breathe.
Instead of taking what has not been offered,
give.

ॐ Honoring Life's Energy: *Brahmacharya*

B*rahmacharya* sometimes translates as honoring God, as well as the rightful use of energy, and often this term is translated to relate to the respectful conduct of sexual energy. This *yama* serves to remind us of the gift and responsibility we have regarding the energy of our life force. We can consider: In what ways do we respect and protect our energies?

Our culture often commends or even congratulates those who work well beyond forty hours per week, which can lead to a desire to prove or earn one's worth through overtaxing the bodily system. However, maintaining a balanced work/rest schedule is a vital part of caring for our well-being through honoring *brahmacharya*. How many hours of sleep we require each night to provide adequate rest for ourselves will vary from person to person, but pushing beyond our capacity will eventually take a toll.

Similarly, we have a choice every time we go to our mat in terms of the intensity of our practice. The types of *āsanas* we choose as well as how long we hold these postures can have effects that are soothing or aggravating to our systems. When we compare ourselves with others, we can enter into a realm of competitive practice, and while it's useful to challenge ourselves to allow for growth, pushing too hard can be counter-productive, resulting in fatigue, aggravation, or injury.

We also have a choice in the mental arena. When we choose to feed our worries, regrets, and fears, we deplete our focus and our reserve of energy. Choosing to bolster our energy in healthy ways through meditation, *prāṇāyāma*, and through realistic, calming thoughts serves to support our energy, honoring the sacred energy we've been given.

Having received a certain amount of stamina or physical strength through genetics, we have a choice to make about how we wish to expend this energy. We can choose to dedicate our creative energies and our general mental, emotional, and physical stamina for the highest good, or we can squander it, intentionally or unintentionally.

Bringing awareness and appreciation to the energy we carry can bring forth our intuitive wisdom, guiding us through the days and nights as we encounter infinite decisions, directing our energy towards what will serve us and those around us best.

ॐ Vitality (*Brahmacharya*)

Is the fuel tank of your energy
half empty or full?

Notice what builds your energy.
Where do you give your energy away?

What depletes you?
What nourishes you?

Draw your energy into center.
Breathe slowly, deeply.
Feel your life force replenishing.

What will you do with this energy?
How will you honor this energy?
This energy, this shining jewel within, is yours.

ॐ Letting Go: *Aparigraha*

A*parigraha* is the *yama* of non-grasping. How often do we feel we need something and then reach to move towards that something? Often the grasp or the reach is internal in the form of longing or trying to make something happen. We may even reach for acknowledgement, for attention, or for things. We may reach without realizing we are reaching, given how conditioned we are to believe that striving is something to be celebrated.

What is enough? When does satisfaction come? When is the amount in the bank account sufficient? When is the level of achievement in the career complete? In all areas of life, there is endless potential for more.

To determine what is necessary or essential is part of this puzzle of *aparigraha*. Is it necessary to have a new car, a new home, a new shirt, or a new phone? Peeling apart the fine layers of want and need can be uncomfortable as we are challenged to come to terms with the truth of our habitual grasping.

Often what we grasp for is security. This is only natural in our mortal realm, and yet it goes against the truth of impermanence. It is a fact that our lives on earth are finite and that nearly everything is bound to change, either subtly or dramatically, and still we resist change, craving a sense of security.

When we realize that all of our outward searching, earnest as it may be, will ultimately leave us empty-handed, we return to the Self and/or to our connection with the Divine. The more regularly and deeply we tap into our inner resources, the less we find we need to grasp.

Breathe into the radiance, the abundance that dwells within.

ॐ Retracting the Reach (*Aparigraha*)

Notice your mind.
If your mind had hands,
how many would be reaching out?
What would they be reaching for?

What grabs for your attention?
What does your attention try to grab?

Return to the center. Return
to the knowing. Return
to the flow of energy within.

Why seek for more
than this moment has to give?
Breathe into it. Receive it fully.
This journey has just begun.

ॐ *Yama Namaskāra*

Oh, ancient five-faceted guide,
knowing us better than we know ourselves,
setting us straight right from the start,
bringing us out of the cave of our self
into the world, vast
with seemingly endless interactions,
you are a *pañchakarma* for our soul,
washing the mind and heart
in a five-step cleanse

On the altar of our best self
you glow, five candles lit:

non-violence, truthfulness,
non-stealing, conservation of energy,
and non-grasping

Daily, we pause. Daily, we embrace
the possibility of keeping
all five candles lit
even as the wind blows
even as the weather shifts
even as we have to re-light
each wick and begin again

Niyama

....

By giving attention to how we are living our life, we can invite shifts in consciousness that can ultimately benefit our psychophysiological well-being. *Niyama*, the second limb of the eight limbs of yoga, is understood to be a set of observances or duties. These are practices that the ancient sages advised for benefit not only in yoga but also in life. Just like yoga poses, these five internal *āsanas*, so to speak, can be deceptively simple; choosing just one to observe for a month, you may begin to see and feel the seemingly endless layers of its depths.

The *niyamas* are:

shaucha

santoṣha

tapas

svādhyāya

Īshvara praṇidhāna.

ॐ Shining Clean: *Shaucha*

I n Āyurveda, the configuration of the internal space of a dwelling is known as *vāstu*. There is an entire science dedicated to understanding the effects of windows, doors, mirrors, and other objects being placed in specific directions (north, south, east, west) in a home or office, much like in the Chinese system of *feng shui*. Think about the relationship between your internal environment and external environment. For instance, consider how you feel when your bedroom or living room is so cluttered that it begins feeling somewhat like an obstacle course. Then, bring to mind how it feels when this room is cleaned, with everything in its rightful place. As our physical surroundings—the rooms, the closets, the drawers, the refrigerator, the yard—come into a state of order and balance, space clears for the clutter inside the mind, the heart, and the body to be cleansed as well.

This internal purification can happen in many ways, including the use of positive affirmations, silent meditation, *prāṇāyāma*, and healthy eating. However, sometimes the "dirt" must first be examined. When we wash our resentments and regrets with forgiveness, the mind and spirit can become quiet and find rest. However, this is usually not an instantaneous process. In fact, it can take quite a while, especially if the residue of conflicted emotions is quite thick from accumulation over time. A house or car that receives regular maintenance can rather easily be cleaned up, but a house or vehicle that has not received attention in a while may involve a multi-step process to bring it back into optimal condition; the same holds true with the vehicle of our body, including all of the intricacies of the mind and spirit as well.

If the task of cleaning up the internal space feels overwhelming or even insurmountable, especially if there may have been substance abuse or other forms of abuse, it may be necessary to ask for support in this process and to take it slowly, one day at a time, keeping in mind that every step taken towards this goal is both valid and valuable.

Start with something that feels doable. Perhaps for one meal a week you choose a healthier option. Maybe the next week it will be two meals, and so on. Similarly, when you first begin there may be just one hour in a day when you do not feed yourself negative thoughts, and then that hour may extend to an hour and a half the next day, and so on.

Little by little, true transformation can happen, but since it often happens so gradually and subtly, the change can be difficult to fully notice and appreciate; keeping a log with even one entry per week can help to foster an accurate and supportive perspective of what is actually taking place and can also become a place where you can acknowledge and celebrate the shifts you are noticing in your environment—both inside and out.

ॐ Removing the Sludge (*Shaucha*)

From the mud, the lotus blooms.
Removing the sludge, there is room.
Room for clarity, room for peace.

Defragment the mind.
Declutter the soul.
Remove debris from the rivers within.

How fresh, how clean is the food,
the water, the music, the interactions
you are feeding yourself daily?

Once the rivers within begin to glisten
with purity, listen.
The entire body begins to sing.

ॐ Embracing Reality: *Santoṣha*

One meaning of *santoṣha* is contentment. How easy is it to be content when we are inundated by images and descriptions of others' lives? When our attention is swept away from the present moment, it can become easy to forget what we appreciate, what we have to be grateful for, such as the breath in our lungs, our ability to see, stand, sit, eat, digest, sleep, smile, and so much more.

Pause for a moment. Think of five things you are thankful for, however big or small as you like. Doing this as a daily practice can be transformative. And you don't have to limit yourself to doing this just once a day. Anytime you start to feel your world get smaller through envy, frustration, or fatigue, pause and bring to mind at least five points of gratitude. Even when something feels impossible, unbearable, or heartbreaking, we can always be thankful that it's not any worse than it already is. To be at peace with what is—how we look, how we feel, our home, our job, our relationships—is no small feat, especially as the dynamics shift from day to day—but with daily awareness, contentment (*santoṣha*) can root and grow.

Consider the trees. Do they resist the turning of their leaves to the colors of autumn? Do they complain that they don't wish to lose their leaves when the weather becomes cool? Do they refuse to allow new growth to emerge in spring? Although the trees don't say a word, we can learn a lot from them about *santoṣha* by simply observing.

For this day, or even this hour, see if you can remain completely content, accepting whatever occurs. And if you can't, see if you can be content with that, too.

ॐ Accepting the Gift of Now (*Santoṣha*)

What if what you already have
is enough?

What if who you already are
is enough?

What if today, with all of its complications,
is just as it is meant to be?

There are changes
we can make today
and others we cannot.

Contentment, with its roots
in acceptance, flowers as we let it.

It does not mean giving up
visions for transformation;
it means accepting what is.
How fully can you embrace
permanence and impermanence?

For this moment, can you release
the past and the future?

Can you accept fully what is—now?

ॐ Alchemy of Change: *Tapas*

Tapas is the fire, or discipline, which allows us to burn through resistance, old patterns of behavior, old habits of thought, and more. It is a potent force that helps us defeat stagnation and move towards our best self. *Tapas* is fire, so it can burn; that is, it can feel intense, but of course two sticks of wood do not transform into glorious flames of light on their own. The trick is keeping *tapas* in balance. We don't ever want to push ourselves so hard that we do harm to ourselves or others; at the same time, *tapas* can keep us from slipping into complacency. By respecting the alchemical properties of *tapas*, we can invite this fire of change into our lives in a way that serves our highest good.

Tapas may take the form of waking up fifteen or thirty minutes earlier so that you can have time to meditate or practice yoga or do *prāṇāyāma* or take a short walk before your daily responsibilities begin. *Tapas* might also mean choosing not to tax your system with sugar or caffeine or highly processed foods. *Tapas* can mean speaking up when it would be easier to stay silent or perhaps staying quiet instead of speaking out of turn. *Tapas* can also mean washing the dishes, doing the laundry, paying the bills on time, remembering to turn your phone off before yoga class begins, and many other manifestations of self-discipline.

So the next time you feel like turning over and going back to sleep instead of rising early; the next time you feel like skipping yoga class; the next time you feel tempted to get fast food or microwave a meal instead of eating something fresh or homemade, place your palm on your navel, your solar plexus, the site of digestive fire, and tap into the alchemy of the heat of transformation that dwells within. By choosing to acknowledge this fire, we can move forward, gently burning through obstacles, cleansing and clearing as we go.

ॐ Shining Brighter (*Tapas*)

When you think you've reached
your limit, take one step more.

Stand straighter. Breathe deeper.

Drop into the deep well
of your resources, reach
into what has always been there,
more than you allowed yourself to believe.

Stretch further,
be stronger, be gentler,
wake up sooner, wake up
fully, be present,
starting now.

Shine in each moment,
brightly, as if it were your last.

ॐ Looking Within: *Svādhyāya*

Svādhyāya is often translated as self-study. What does it mean to study the self? Often we associate the word "study" with school—with study guides, quizzes, and exams. This may be a positive or negative association, depending upon our experience. However, *svādhyāya* moves beyond study in an institution or formal structure and welcomes the study of spiritual texts and one's self, inviting the practices of observation, awareness, and reflection to flourish.

For example, by placing our attention on specific regions of the body, such as the abdomen, the back of the knee, and the inner elbow, we can soften into a deeper awareness of the nuances of the miracles of our anatomy and physiology, learning to stay within our body rather than escaping to our minds or to various habits or substances.

Our minds, behaviors, and habits can be a little more challenging to observe, especially when the mind can be swayed by illusions, mistaking them for truth. One way to still the mind is through meditation. This can be formal meditation, sitting quietly while following the breath, or it can be a walking meditation or even meditation coming through a creative process like composing music or artwork.

Additionally, it can be helpful to record observations of yourself, such as in a daily log or chart of your own design. This way you can begin to notice patterns that may emerge from week to week, month to month.

Freewriting can also be an effective way to observe the thoughts and emotions that are occupying space and energy. Freewriting is exactly what it sounds like—writing freely, not pausing to correct a spelling mistake or to overanalyze. In fact, the main guideline is that you write for a specific period of time without stopping. In the beginning, you might try writing for five minutes per day. You might later expand this to a ten-minute session, or perhaps try five minutes when you wake up and five minutes before you go to sleep at night. This can allow you to take inventory of your intentions for the day in the morning and then reflect upon them at the end of the day.

Essentially, when we are looking at our life as a painting or as a film, we can slow down and pause, even zoom in or rewind, to consider more closely what we said, how we said it, why we said it, and, if given the chance again, if we would make any changes. This same approach can be used to reflect upon our written words, our actions, and our interactions. The idea is not to criticize ourselves but to be honest and attentive, allowing self-awareness to flourish.

ॐ Who Are You? (*Svādhyāya*)

Who are you?
Who is the one
sitting inside of you
listening, watching,
feeling?

What do you feel?
Where do you feel it?
What do your eyes notice
as they observe the world,
as they look within?

Who are your parents,
your ancestors?
Where did you come from?
Where are you headed?
What is your goal?

Who are you right now?
How does your body
align with your mind
and with your soul?

Who are you in silence?
Who are you in sound?
Who are you in motion?
Who are you when you are still?

What is your relationship
to earth, water, fire, air, space,
to the sun, moon, stars,
with animals and plants,
with buildings and computers and cars,
with each other,
with your Self?

ॐ Opening to Grace:
Īshvara Praṇidhāna

One of the translations of *Īshvara praṇidhāna* is surrendering to the Divine, which may sound, depending upon your point of view, as a beautiful or painful process. "Surrender" can take on questionable connotations when its synonyms are considered: yield, relent, give in, submit, cave in, capitulate, acquiesce, and yet "surrender" has a range of meanings that offer more possibilities for interpreting and understanding. Letting go, which is sometimes looked down upon in a society that often prides itself on workaholism and a 24/7 routine, can actually bring forth a sense of peace, liberation, balance, and well-being through loosening our grip on our attachments.

Bring to mind a list of the top ten things you feel you could not live without. Was your cell phone on that list? If it was, surrendering does not mean giving away your phone or disconnecting the service. Instead, it may mean putting your phone in silent mode for a period of time during the day, increasing the length of time as you feel able. It might mean choosing several times a day to engage in texting, emailing, or listening to voicemails rather than having messaging taking place from the moment you wake until the moment you sleep. It might simply mean allowing yourself to do your morning practices before checking your phone or email, or some other modification that works for you.

Īshvara praṇidhāna involves faith. Just as we must have faith that setting the phone aside for a few moments or a few hours will be bearable, *Īshvara praṇidhāna* challenges us to have faith in the divinity of how events are unfolding. This can be especially challenging when the events feel like errors or injustices. "Why now?" we may ask, or "Why me?" These questions can bring a maze-like torment as we seek to understand what is not available for us to understand. However, if we have faith in the divine wisdom that is knitting our lives together with unseen threads, we can more readily accept the current reality, reducing our suffering.

To receive a taste of *Īshvara praṇidhāna*, select just one situation that has recently been circling through your consciousness, perhaps bringing undue suffering through a sense that things are not as they should be. Feel all of the frustration and upset that this situation represents to you (perhaps clenching your muscles tightly), and then let it go. *Siṃhāsana* (Lion Pose) can be helpful here. Allow the tightness you feel around this issue to soften by breathing into it, accepting that this situation has a perfect place within the divine choreography of life, and that this will become more apparent at some point in the future. Breathe. The sky did not fall. You did not collapse. You are honoring a sacred *niyama*. Breathe.

ॐ Faith in the Unseen (*Īshvara Praṇidhāna*)

Let go. Lay down your fears, your anger,
your worries, your doubts, your despair.

Can you trust the unseen calligraphy
writing the script of this day?

On the altar of your heart
let fragrant flowers rest
with soft candles illuminating
rich offerings of faith.

Sitting with palms facing up,
open to receive,
feel the grace of the divine.

Sitting with palms facing up,
surrender, relinquishing
any need or expectation
to receive.

Sitting with palms facing up,
breathe, every breath
filling us, illuminating us,
our rawest, emptiest places
transmuting into light.

ॐ *Niyama Namaskāra*

You,
five windows shining
into our heart, not allowing us to hide,
your dimensions wide, inviting the light
to pour in
so that we look, not just look,
but see our Self and observe:

how clean we are (body, soul, and mind),
how content we are
(regardless of the vicissitudes of life),
how much self-discipline we have
for positive transformation,
how often and how deeply we reflect on our own self,
and how fully we surrender,
placing our vulnerability and faith
in the arms of the Divine

Niyama, you humble us
with your simplicity
that is not so simple at all.
We raise the blinds,
open the curtains
of each of your five windows
and see smudges
where our attention has drifted away.
We breathe. We notice,
accepting both the smudges and the shine,
trusting the divine architecture
of this moment, this breath.

Āsana

....

Āsanas are the physical postures of yoga.

ॐ Oceanic Depths

W hen you think of yoga, do you think primarily of being "on the mat"? *Āsana*, the third limb of yoga, focuses on the physical postures. Some of these poses resemble aspects of nature, such as *Tāḍāsana* (Mountain Pose), or *Ardha Chandrāsana* (Half-Moon), whereas some resemble animals, such as *Adho Mukha Shvānāsana* (Downward Dog), or *Shalabhāsana* (Locust). Still others resemble objects or shapes, such as *Setu Bandha Sarvāngāsana* (Bridge) or *Trikoṇāsana* (Triangle). By moving the body into these positions, we stretch and strengthen. The activation of acupressure points (*marma* points) on the body through *āsana* has therapeutic effects on the psychophysiological system as well.

Āsana can be as simple as standing in *Tāḍāsana* (Mountain), or as complex as standing in *Tāḍāsana* with full awareness of the four corners of the soles of the feet, the alignment of the ankles, hips, shoulders, and spine, while breathing slowly, deeply, and evenly, fully relaxed and aware simultaneously. Similarly, each *āsana* has oceanic depths. They reveal themselves when we enter into *āsana* fresh, with a beginner's mind, even as we meet the poses with the familiarity of longtime friends.

Just as we could spend our life (or perhaps several lifetimes) trying to learn as many *āsanas* as possible or exploring each of the different styles of *āsana*, such as *vinyāsa, yin, haṭha*, and others, we could also spend our entire life diving deeper into the *āsanas* that we know already, seeking to open ourselves to the depths—the subtle nuances—of the layers of each posture that arise when we can acknowledge that even in our practiced skill, we are still at the shore, and bow with reverence to the vast unknown.

ॐ Entering the *Āsana*

Each time we enter into *āsana*, we have a choice of how we do so. We can do so mechanically, as if we were on autopilot. We can do so with stress and strain, pushing to match an image of the pose from a book or magazine, or we can stay close to the breath, remaining present with what is emerging within us, physically, mentally, and emotionally, as we go deeper into the pose.

We can also consider the nature of the pose, layer by layer, approaching the pose as a beginner entering it for the very first time, listening to every cue carefully as if it is vital information, feeling every sensation in our body, noticing every nuance.

When we enter *Garuḍāsana*, for instance, are we becoming the eagle, or are we just configuring ourselves in a specific way? Can we become the Mountain, the Locust, the Dancer, the Bridge, the Warrior? If not, what is stopping us?

ॐ Consider the Moon

Sometimes our schedules may not allow us to attend yoga class on a regular basis; there may even be a challenge to find time to do a full home practice. This often leads to completely giving up on doing yoga. However, what if you were to do a single *āsana*? Practicing a single *āsana* allows a savoring of its properties. When we eat an entire meal, we do not always notice the individual flavors and textures of all the components. Yet when we eat a piece of fruit or dessert by itself, we can fully experience its sweetness. Similarly, we can do so many *āsanas* within a class that we may not be able to remember them all even an hour afterwards. When the body receives just one *āsana*, the opportunity for experiencing it deeply is present in a new way.

Consider the moon. It is up there every night, whether we notice it or not. We might see it in our peripheral vision as we hurry on our journey. But how often do we actually sit and observe the moon? How often do we consider the half-moon? Do we even think of it when we are in *Ardha Chandrāsana* (Half-Moon Pose)? In what ways do the phases of the moon inhabit our practice, as our dedication and devotion waxes and wanes? In what ways are we more or less observant than we might think?

ॐ Wealth

What is wealth? Wealth can certainly be measured in terms of dollars or even property and possessions; however, there is also a wealth of health, having the energy and stamina to partake in the activities of life without struggle or strain. Yet, just as there can be good physical health without corresponding mental and emotional well-being, true riches come, metaphorically, when there is equanimity of body, mind, and spirit.

Wealth can also appear in the form of beauty, such as the blessing of a sunrise brilliant with bright pink and orange, an ocean wave reflecting the light of the moon, or a field of wild sunflowers.

The wealth of each day can be measured differently. When we take account of what brings us comfort, what brings us joy, and what brings us inspiration, we have a sense of whether individual experiences have brought us to a greater sense of appreciation, or whether there has been a sense of depletion. Consider yesterday. Was it a day of wealth, a day of poverty, or somewhere in between? Although we cannot always alter the balance in our bank account, we can often influence the prosperity of our attitude and spirit. Each time we enter into a yogic practice we tap into an inner health, an inner wealth, one that may not be fully measured but one that can be felt. As we observe the riches of each *āsana*, we enter a wealth that resides at our core, shining like a golden coin.

ॐ To Flow or Not to Flow

When was the last time you were so focused on what you were doing that you lost track of time? When we are in a flow, we often lose track of the hours in the joy that comes from synchronicity or alignment with our true nature. Aligning with your true nature may mean cooking, running, singing, designing buildings, or something else entirely. By communing with our true nature, we can envision what we genuinely have to offer to the community. When we are doing what we were born to do, and what brings radiance to our hearts, we are at our best and generate an energy that can fuel our efforts in a sustainable way. Sometimes what we were born to do is very clear to us and other times it can seem more like a mystery. Often, by doing things and realizing that they are not enjoyable we can more easily understand, in contrast, what we *do* enjoy. Sometimes by simply observing someone who is within the flow we can feel what it means to be free.

As you move through your next *āsana* practice or even as you move through your day, notice when there is an almost effortless flow when events are happening naturally with ease, as well as where there seems to be obstruction to fluidity. Breathe. Is your breath flowing? Listen to it. Follow it. Synchronize with its rhythm of in-breath, out-breath, in-breath, out-breath. What would it take to bring this flow into your day?

ॐ Finding the Balance

I n Half-Moon, in Warrior 3, in Tree Pose, what happens in your mind when your body wobbles, when your balance wavers? Does your mind respond critically? Do you immediately try to correct or erase the imbalance? Next time you feel that instability, stay with it, observing it. By immediately reacting, we often overcorrect, missing the experience of what we can learn from being within the imbalance.

Our lives repeatedly offer us balancing poses as we decide what to eat and how much to eat, how often and how intensely to practice, how many hours to work and sleep, how much time to spend indoors versus outdoors, how much money to spend or save, how much to speak or stay in silence, how active or passive to be in any given situation, and the list goes on.

Rather than jumping from one extreme to the other, when we can stay with the uncertainty, observing our position, whether in an actual balancing pose or within one of the continuums of life, we can begin to make micro-movements, noticing the effects of our gradual repositioning, finding our center, steadily moving into a balance we can sustain.

ॐ Life as a Prism

What was your life like ten years ago, twenty years ago? Do the same songs, activities, foods, and beliefs carry the exact same importance? In some cases, the answer may be "yes," but in many cases subtle or tremendous transformations may have occurred. There may have even been a change of job, career, living space, and/or relationship. In this sense, we can experience many "lives" within a single lifetime; in fact, if you have ever cleaned out a storage unit, or even a closet or attic or basement, and come across memorabilia from decades past, you likely have a good sense of this phenomenon.

If you were to name five "lives" that you've had in this lifetime, what would they be? Which ones did you cherish the most? Which lives have you yet to lead? Pausing to look back every five years or so can yield motivation for change as well as reflection and appreciation for what has been experienced in this swiftly moving magnificent life. Even a single day can seem to contain multiple layers as we change roles and circumstances.

The next time you move into *āsana*, see how many layers of sensation you can observe in your body, noticing also the layers of the mind as it recalls how you have inhabited the pose previously and imagines how you might do this pose in the future. Then, see what it takes to bring yourself back to the present, aware of the many layers but not clinging to any of them, accepting your pose and accepting yourself just as you are right now.

ॐ Centering

72,000 *nāḍīs*, energy pathways
spreading like rivers through us

the navel echoing the wordlessness of the womb,
our connection to what came before, the long months
when we, like the gentlest of mercies, were carried

mystical portal,
circling back to our beginnings,
the center song in us
softening, if we let it,
its tightness blossoming gently
into a *maṇḍala* of light

ॐ Impermanence

The concept of impermanence is so much easier to accept when it is just a concept. When impermanence marches into our life, however, in the loss of a loved one, a job, health, or some other central aspect, the impact is profound. There can be an inward collapse, as well as a wide array of emotions, ranging from shock and disbelief to anger and rage, to sorrow, depression, and confusion. Mentally we may understand, for instance, that every human being must die. After all, there are few towns or cities without large cemeteries displaying the many lives that have come to an end. We may have even attended several funerals and burials, yet there can still be something in the soul that subconsciously yearns to believe that this fate will somehow be spared for a loved one.

Impermanence, though, is with us always. The moment that existed when you first began this meditation is gone, absolutely finished. There may be an echo, a memory, a resonance from this moment, but the moment itself is gone. Moment by moment, we expire. And yet with life's momentum, we are propelled continually forward, making it easy for us to forget the delicacy, the vulnerability, the sacredness of the present moment.

It is within meditation, within slowing down, that we can reconnect with our breath, and become aware again of the present moment. As you rest in *Shavāsana* after your next yoga practice, as you breathe into each moment, do so with the awareness of each moment dissolving, never to be lived again. Inhale slowly. Exhale even more slowly. Can you feel the fragility, the sacredness, the beauty, the singularity of this once-in-a-lifetime moment?

ॐ Surface vs. Depth

The surface of the sea dances in sunlight, the flowing waves glittering like jewels. The same surface on a cloudy day may turn a dull gray. Regardless of shifts in weather, the appearance of the surface may not match the contents of the sea. A sparkling surface may belie toxins and debris floating beneath. A slate gray surface may obscure treasures below. The presence of bright yellow and blue fish or large sea turtles moving in a relaxed underwater ballet may be hidden from sight.

Similarly, there is a surface of every *āsana*, and then there are the varying layers of depth of the pose. A pose that may gleam on the surface in terms of looking beautiful and correct may not be the full pose if, for instance, the breathing is not full and deep, or if the mind is elsewhere, or has become a stormy sea. Conversely, a pose that is far from picture-perfect may harbor the treasure of authentic practice if body, breath, and consciousness are working together.

What is the texture and appearance of the surface of this moment? Are you ready to breathe into what exists beneath?

ॐ The Pause

I mages on the covers of yoga magazines that look back at us while we wait to check out at the grocery store are often dynamic *āsanas*—*āsanas* that are beautiful to observe and difficult to do. In the extraordinary array of yoga *āsanas* that exist, attention is often drawn to the complexity and magnificence of balancing poses like *Naṭarājāsana* (Dancer Pose), *Shīrṣhāsana* (Headstand), or *Kākāsana* (Crow Pose). And yet, lying on our back with the knees hugged into the chest, *Pawanmuktāsana/Apānāsana* (Knees-to-Chest), renowned for supporting digestion, is a potent pose, just as the more dramatic poses that are often showcased. According to Āyurveda, the health of digestive fire (*agni*) is a primary factor in overall health. Therefore, taking time to practice Knees-to-Chest on a regular basis may significantly transform a life.

Similarly, taking time to observe the pauses in life can change our perspective. Silences, whether fleeting or sustained, have significance. We can speed right past these silent pauses, disregarding them, or we can consider them as equally important or even more important than sound. Consider music. What would the layers of the ocean of music be without the carefully placed rests? In the music of your own life, where are the pauses? Are they abrupt and resented, planned and accepted, or spontaneously enjoyed?

As you move into your next *āsana* practice, be aware not only of the poses but also the pauses between them. Just as there is a *vipāka*, or post-digestive effect of the foods we eat, there is a post-digestive effect of each *āsana* as our bodies and minds receive its nourishment. As we pause between poses, we allow ourselves to receive the full effects—mind, body, spirit—of each pose, and we allow ourselves to recalibrate, returning to center.

ॐ Inverting the View

What do you see when your head hangs upside down in a Standing Straddle Forward Fold (*Prasārita Pādottānāsana*)? As the crown of your head faces the earth, neck and head relaxing, the ceiling is now the floor.

Just as we may have to refresh the screen when we are working online, inverting our position, literally, can refresh our view, our perspective.

It's easy to get locked into a standpoint on an issue, and maintaining this position, such as surrounding ourselves with those who share similar backgrounds and beliefs, only reinforces it. By turning upside down, even partially, we turn the tables, giving our systems a chance to refresh and reboot.

Take a situation that you feel very strongly about and stand it on its head. Believe for a moment that you feel exactly the opposite. Allow yourself to soften into this belief as if it were your own, as if the floor has become the ceiling. Explore this reality as fully and genuinely as possible. Just as the body signals to us to come up when we've been in an inversion long enough, you will feel when you have had your fill of this opposing view. By acknowledging yes and no, up and down, inner and outer, false and true, the full picture begins to come into view.

ॐ Body of Prayer

Within the sacred temple of this day
each posture breathes a holy prayer
scripting the calligraphy
of each moment in gold

Each posture, a living breathing way
to say: I, head to toe, am alive,
and whatever else may not be working,
breath is flowing through me
beautifully,

I can choose to smile or grimace
or to keep my features calm,
each posture an expression
of my gratitude, my devotion,
eloquent in stillness,
in motion, gazing softly,

offering my practice
with reverence, with intention,
with authenticity, alive
to each and every moment,
each sacred breath

ॐ Warrior 1

To enter into *Vīrabhadrāsana I* (Warrior 1), we step one foot forward. We can lurch forward haphazardly, or we can move mindfully from our center. As we lift our arms and bend the front knee, we are simultaneously in a position of vulnerability and victory. Our chest is exposed, and our heart can open, while the bending knee puts us in a courageous position to advance as needed. This simultaneous combining of opposing forces brings us more keenly alive to the present moment. We breathe courage in; we breathe fear out.

What situation in your life is one that you have been avoiding, either directly or indirectly? What would it take for you to look—really look—at this situation? As you move into Warrior 1, envision this person, place, emotion, thought, or situation of challenge standing before you. Instead of trying to conquer or vanquish the opposition, focus on your breathing. Focus on truly looking, both at what is in front of you and what you are feeling within. Stay with the pose as long as you can comfortably, and then take several more breaths, moving gently beyond your perceived limit. Afterwards, return to standing, to *Tāḍāsana* (Mountain Pose), again, noticing what you feel, both physically and within the emotional body. What would it take to face this challenge with courage, with compassion, with patience, with strength, with love?

ॐ Warrior 2

As a warrior, awareness is vital. A warrior must be able to hear and observe keenly in a 360-degree radius. Timing is essential as well. Moving, or choosing not to move, a second too soon or a second too late, can have dire consequences, and yet a warrior must remain deeply calm. While a warrior may be born with a propensity to some of these qualities, dedicated training is also needed. Similarly, our ability to move gracefully and effectively in and out of conflicts requires practice and training.

We can practice this process on our mat as we move into *Vīrabhadrāsana II* (Warrior 2). As we take a wide stance, lower the hips, and bend the front knee, we extend the arms, opening our heart. Even as we turn our head and gaze over the front fingertips, our right and left fingertips reach out in opposite directions. As we extend the front arm towards all that may appear on our path, the back arm points to previous conflicts we may have experienced.

What does it feel like to stay in this position, facing a challenge head-on? Can you stand steadily and with grace with full awareness of the conflict? Breathe. Notice any quickening or slowing of the heartbeat.

As you come to back to center, pause. Breathe. As you change sides and move into the pose facing the opposite direction, notice what feels different and what feels the same. See how alert you can stay without tightening your shoulders, your forehead, your jaw. Breathe.

Go into the pose once more. This time as you turn to gaze over your fingertips, bring to your consciousness a conflict that resides within your own thoughts and emotions. Then, as you switch sides, bring to mind a conflict that exists outside of yourself with another person or out in the world. Breathe in your strength. Breathe out your fear.

Sometimes we can anticipate when we will meet conflicts or challenges, and sometimes they appear suddenly. As we train ourselves in the unification of body, mind, and spirit through yoga, we prepare ourselves for those moments when we need to stand up for ourselves or for someone or something. Cultivating both strength and gentleness, as well as awareness, we can redefine what it means to be, with the utmost integrity, a warrior for peace, for justice, for compassion, for love.

ॐ Warrior 3

Often war is thought of as a contest to see who will be victorious; however, victory can be defined in very different ways, especially when it comes to losses and gains, both tangible and intangible. War can bring to mind the capture of property, funds, objects, and even human lives, and yet if we redefine loss and success, success may become more about letting go than accumulating.

Vīrabhadrāsana III (Warrior 3) is a pose that symbolizes the challenge and necessity of letting go. In this pose, where we are virtually suspended in the air, we must find balance and strength as we root down into the standing leg.

Where is the heavy armor in a pose like this? Rather than barricading ourselves in what we think may protect us, we focus, ground, lift, and extend, reaching into space, rooting into faith.

Warrior 3 can feel a bit like being a bird in flight. There are birds of prey and birds of song. Some are one and the same. Similarly, there are many types of warriors, and a single warrior can have many different stances. Bring to mind what you feel like when you are in Warrior 1 and then revisit what you feel like in Warrior 2 and Warrior 3. If we approach each conflict the same exact way, we can intensify the conflict; however, by recognizing the unique nature of each challenge we encounter, we can move into each one with awareness and grace.

ॐ Mountain

The mountains loom large, shaping the horizon. They are silently bold, standing tall in the face of any weather, any political upheaval, any epidemic. Carrying the sun and moon on their backs, they do not waver; they do not crumble or fall. Steady in the fiercest of winds, they keep their center, witnessing all of the beauty and chaos in the surrounding lands. They are wise in their silence, observing what changes and what does not change, one millennium to the next.

When we stand in Mountain Pose, *Tāḍāsana*, what do we embody of the strength and stability of the mountains? Do our feet press firmly into the ground, weight equally distributed on the four corners of the soles of our feet? Are our ankles, hips, and shoulders aligned? Does our head rest at the top of our spine, neither leaning forward nor backward but in steady alignment?

Mountain Pose, in its seeming simplicity, can perhaps seem like it's not an *āsana*, and yet when we fully engage our awareness of the breath and the body, feeling every facet from the soles of the feet to the crown of the head, we become part of something as ancient, majestic, and humbling as the mountains, standing firmly in the presence of Self.

ॐ Tree

Are trees sentient beings? It depends whom you ask. Year by year, with the rings of their trunks expanding, their height increasing, the reach of their branches stretching further, they are an undeniable presence in the landscape of our lives. If there is a tree that has grown by your home for many years, it may even feel like part of the family.

As familiar as trees are, how much do we really understand about them? Just as a cardiologist can devote decades of study to the heart and find that a full understanding of this central vessel is elusive, so too can a botanist devote a lifetime to these trunked beings and still not reach a complete understanding. Palm trees, pine trees, banyan trees, neem trees, magnolia trees, dogwoods, juniper, bonsai trees, weeping willows, maples, oaks, tulip poplars, birch trees—if you were a tree, which one would you be? Would you be a sapling, an aged tree, one that's been struck by lightning, one that harbors nests of singing birds, a symmetrical tree, one that sways in the wind?

As you become that tree, feel the roots pushing out from the soles of your feet through the floor and into the earth, reaching three feet, and then ten feet, both outward and down. What feeds the tree of you? What do you need most in your life? Are you rooting into it now? Notice if you feel nourished or if your roots thirst, seeking for something known or unknown. You are a tree, and you are strong. You will weather many seasons of the soul; you already have.

ॐ Child

There are certain features of this life that are universal, such as sun, earth, and sky. We also, no matter where we live, share the experience of living within the architecture of bone and breath. Similarly, we have all had the experience of being a child.

Bālāsana (Child's Pose) asks us to rest our forehead gently on Mother Earth, to relinquish our need to be a Mountain, a Warrior, or anything else. Relaxing in this position, we soothe the nervous system. Arms may reach forward on the floor beyond the head, or they may drop back along the sides of the body towards the feet.

This is a posture of surrendering, letting go. There are many ways in which adult life necessitates being alert and responsible, and while each period of life has its own expectations and goals, sometimes as adults we can become hypervigilant and overwork ourselves.

Bālāsana is a time to relax, let go, giving into the very natural human need for comfort and support. Childhood is also often a time of imagination, possibility, play, and fun. Do these elements still have space to breathe in your life? If not, how might you let them feel more welcome? For now, just rest. Breathe.

We are all somebody's child. We are all children of the universe. Although we may be fully grown in terms of height, we are all still growing and changing within. When we can feel gratitude for our safe passage into this world and the elements that carried us through our early years, we can honor our past, with awareness of both its challenges and its gifts...and embrace more fully the present now.

ॐ Corpse Pose

"*S*havāsana" is a word that flows, rolling off the tongue, bringing to mind a deep relaxation. And yet hearing the English translation, Corpse Pose, may have quite a different effect. However, thinking of *Shavāsana* as Corpse Pose can help us understand why this seemingly simple pose (just resting on your back without "doing" anything) can feel so difficult.

Are we ready to die? Are the things we are dedicating our life to valuable and potent enough to comfort us at the time of death? Will our professional accomplishments or our bank accounts or our social media accounts offer comfort? Or will it be our loved ones? What if our loved ones are not able to be present? What within ourselves will we be able to draw upon? If we have practiced regularly with finding peace in our breath, especially in Corpse Pose, will we draw from this well of inner peace when the time comes for us to exit our bodies?

When we attempt to lie still in Corpse Pose, the body or mind will likely resist. There may be an itch, a place of discomfort in the body, a tremor, a shaking, a question, a worry, a problem to solve that arises in the mind. The mind is very clever and may try to convince us that this is a perfect time to sort through our thoughts since we're not "doing" anything else anyway. However, when we can bypass this chatter, we can enter into deep relaxation. Forcefully bypassing does not tend to work, but gently acknowledging our thought pattern and returning to the breath can allow these stirred-up waves in the mental ocean to eventually settle.

Exploring any anxiety that you have about accepting the inevitability of death may be useful. Is there something you have not yet said or done that you could work on to bring yourself to a greater readiness or acceptance, even if death is a long way off?

When entering into *Shavāsana* at the end of class, see how much you can let go—allowing the floor to support you, allowing your mind to empty, allowing the body and breath to soften and slow. As our nervous system and muscular system relax, we rest, immersed within the permanent impermanence of our lives.

Embodying the Poses

Sometimes we can move almost mechanically into *āsana*, especially if it is a familiar pose that we have done hundreds of times before. If we focus solely on the muscles of the body or if we allow the mind to drift to what we need to buy at the grocery store or the email or text we need to write, or any number of other topics, we can miss part of the pose.

Staying connected to the breath helps to unite the mind and body. Similarly, reading or listening to an *āsana* meditation prior to moving into the pose—or listening to it during an extended hold—may take you deeper into the pose.

After trying some of the *āsana* meditations that follow, see if you might like to create some of your own to explore.

ॐ Mountain (*Tāḍāsana*)

The mountain in you remains strong.
The mountain in you does not flinch.
The mountain in you does not collapse
even as storms rush through.
The mountain in you does not forget
how you arose from the ground.
The mountain in you remembers
what has been mined and what remains.
The mountain in you holds nightly *satsaṅg*
with the stars and the moon.
The mountain in you feels the softness
of the clouds as they pass by.
The mountain in you holds
many secrets you may never tell.
The mountain in you harbors dragonflies and hawks
as freely as it harbors ants, panthers, and snakes.
The mountain in you becomes prayer
as the sun rises out of dawn.
The mountain in you will, in the end,
return to its foundations, unshaken.
The mountain in you is the part of you
the world cannot break.
The mountain in you, when it breathes
into its truth, stops others in its tracks.
The mountain in you, from first breath
to last, the mountain, the divine mountain
in you—is *you.*

ॐ Child (*Bālāsana*)

Kneeling, forehead to the ground,
arms outstretched before you,
hips to heels, spine long,
palms into the earth,
you, the innocent child,
surrendering the posturing
of an adult,
letting go of the need
to be a mountain, warrior,
dancer, lion, boat,
or anything other
than what you are,
surrendering your sorrow,
your anger, your fear,
your boredom, your confusion,
breathing into the wonder
of a child gazing up
for the first time
at the immense luminosity
of the moon

ॐ Boat (*Nāvāsana*)

Legs and arms lifting, extending,
spine long, chest expanding,
you, a boat able to find its way
through the most challenging
storms of this life,
you, a boat navigating
through the surging
thoughts and emotions
arising within,
you, a boat, guided
by constellations
of your internal GPS,
steered by the depth
of your faith,
the clarity of your vision,
even when night clouds come
obscuring the stars and moon

ॐ Bound Angle (*Baddha Koṇāsana*)

Sitting with spine long
knees widening
soles of the feet
coming together
like hands pressed in prayer.
Opening the feet gently
as if opening a book—
the book of your life,
written in the lines
on the soles of your feet,
the palms of your hands,
your face, the story
of your life written
with each breath,
each decision and indecision,
each action and inaction,
each word, each silence,
each and every pause,
each scene on the stage
in the *līlā*, the play of life,
spilling into the next,
word by moment by breath

ॐ Bridge (*Setu Bandha Sarvāṅgāsana*)

You, the bridge between your body and mind
You, the bridge between your mind and soul
You, the bridge between your ancestors and all you create
You, the bridge between no and yes, right and wrong
You, the bridge between grudge and forgive
You, the bridge between despair and hope
You, the bridge between sleep and dream
You, the bridge between forget and renew
You, with your spine's arc lifting beautifully to the sky
You, the bridge between past and future
You, the bridge crossing the ocean of now

ॐ Dancer (*Naṭarājāsana*)

You, balancing beautifully,
you, with your stationary dance,
moving without moving,
your grace, your calmness,
your fluidity, your strength,
the way you inhabit your body—
fully—completely—
your presence on this earth
an ongoing gift, a dance,
a prayer without words,
you, dancer, dancing with each
micro-movement of your stance,
your thoughts, your emotions,
the ever-evolving choreography
in life's exquisite dance

ॐ Downward Dog (*Adho Mukha Shvānāsana*)

Your body in an upside-down V,
tailbone lifting up to the sky,
palms of the hands and soles of the feet
pressing into the ground,
fingers and toes spread,
legs and arms strong,
you, in this moment, a four-footed being,
your mouth beyond the reach of speech,
your senses alive, alert to every sound,
every movement and scent,
the nuanced language
of observation and intuition
coursing through your spine.

ॐ Forward Fold (*Uttānāsana*)

Arms lifting overhead,
standing tall,
hinging at the hips,
feet rooting into the ground,
crown of the head
releasing towards the floor,
chest pressing in towards the thighs,
the body folding in half
neatly like a suitcase

What are you carrying?
Which thoughts bulge
against the seams of your mind?

Letting go, relax your mind,
the strength of your legs
supporting you,
extraneous thoughts
spilling out the top of your head
releasing softly into the ground

ॐ Half-Moon
(*Ardha Chandrāsana*)

The middle point
between full moon and new moon,
you, carrying both the light and the night,
you, luminous, the still point
between waxing and waning,
you, with the wisdom
of the lunar cycle
conducting the oceanic tides,
the music of the depths
following your lead,
you, appearing and disappearing,
regular in your rhythm,
bold in your light pouring forth
commingling with the black hole of night
as easily as with the dreams of the stars

ॐ Knees-to-Chest (*Apānāsana*)

You, resting on your back,
wrapping your arms
around your knees,
hugging yourself,
hugging your struggles,
your pains, your sorrows,
hugging your mistakes
with the softest compassion,
exhaling them out,
hugging your beauty,
strength, originality, and joy,
feeling your backbone resting on the floor,
feeling your chest rise and fall,
feeling your arms
encircling you,
your practice,
this moment,
and you
a flower bud
just about to bloom

ॐ Lion (*Siṃhāsana*)

You, body of courage,
your mouth wide,
tongue extending,
breath expanding,
your exhale roaring
from deep within,
your hands, sharply clawed,
raised in front of you,
your eyes wide, full of light,
gazing upward,
and you, sitting on your haunches,
ready to spring, yet
perfectly calm, still,
your full intensity rising,
charging your throat,
exhaling completely,
inhaling strength
into every molecule,
your being brimming
with life, a continuous flow
of wild sweet strength
clearing the
path before you

ॐ Tree (*Vṛkṣhāsana*)

Standing firm as a trunk
rooted securely, deeply—
your breath, your mind expanding
like the branches of a tree,
thoughts fluttering like leaves
in a gentle breeze,
then becoming still, serene,
a silent witness, even as weather shifts,
bending, swaying as the winds arise
and the storms surge through,
you, centered; you, sturdy at your core
you, feeling the support of the earth
and all that nourishes you,
your roots reaching deeper,
you, serene; you, moving with the wind
you, a landmark,
you, a shelter,
you, beautiful and strong
in your unique design,
you, wise without words,
you, born of sun and moon,
rain and stars,
wind and earth,
your expanding branches
mirroring
a labyrinth of roots below

ॐ Triangle (*Trikoṇāsana*)

Past, present, future.
Morning, noon, night.

Three-part harmonies
braiding through:
compassion, clarity, commitment
devotion, discipline, direction
beauty, balance, blessing.

Look at the triangle
your legs make with the earth.
Feel the triangle from arms to legs to floor,
from shoulder blades to sacrum.

Observe the triangles
in your day-to-day relations:
I-me-my; he-she-you; you-they-us

Yesterday, today, tomorrow.
Sun, moon, stars.
Yes, no, maybe.
Breath, bone, blood.
Body, spirit, mind.
Feet, navel, crown.

City, state, nation.
Country, continent, globe.

In the triangle
of *was, is, will be*
of body, spirit and mind,
find the center,
breathe into the now.

ॐ Warrior (*Vīrabhadrāsana*)

You, standing strong in Self,
you, looking straight ahead,
looking into the present moment,
accepting the truth
of your mind, your heart,
not looking away,
breathing into the discomfort,
breathing into the comfort
of you, your authentic self,
your chest expanding,
your heart shining,
full of compassion and courage,
ready to confront,
to embrace, face
whatever challenge
arrives in front of you
next

ॐ *Shavāsana*

The muscles deep within the thigh
protest. The chin, tucked, neck extending,
stretches the brain stem where who knows what
begins to stir. Decades waking up find themselves
out of order and not sure where they stand.
Out of the spaces between vertebrae
hatch small dinosaurs with surprisingly large
teeth. Half of them want to pray and chant;
the other half are predators searching for prey.
A cosmos of planets and stars swirls
at the throat, the moon of the heart
waxing and waning. Up through the blue
veins that are not so much blue
as they are the long "moo" of a lone cow
on the plains swim iridescent whales
spouting generations memorized in verse.
Tides, governed by the heart's moon,
ebb and flow. The palms, symmetrical,
find that the lines on the left map
don't match the ones on the right.
The hip bones from the depths
of their sockets proclaim
it doesn't matter if the symmetrical
is asymmetrical now and then,
the eyes in their orbital sockets
roll and then soften, the antennae
of the fingertips and toe tips let go,
the jaw unclenches, the breath becoming
increasingly slow and quiet,
nearly imperceptible,
the bones themselves dissipating
into the cavernous black hole of now.

ॐ Corpse Pose (*Shavāsana*)

To die to each day, moment, word, breath.
The rosewater scent fading away.
The sky giving up its blue.
Somewhere, geese soaring home.
Petals releasing, imperceptibly.
Translucent opalescence of all
that once was, is, will someday be.
The faintest whisper. Shimmering.
Lifting up like mist, all that once contained.

ॐ Meditative Movement

Repeating a brief meditative phrase silently or aloud during *āsana* can take us deeper into a pose, allowing us to embody it more fully—body, mind, and spirit. After reading the meditative *āsana* phrases below, perhaps you may wish to create some of your own, expressing your practice from the inside out.

Boat: I navigate the changing currents of life with confidence and ease.

Bound Angle: My feet open like the book of my life, written with every step, every breath.

Bow: I am a bow through which the sweetest arrow of silence may sing.

Bridge: As my spine arches, I bridge *was* with *will be*.

Camel: I drop back into that which I cannot see with the faith of one who has crossed the desert blind.

Chair: I sit with stability and ease in the center of my strength.

Child: Relaxing, releasing, I surrender to Mother Earth, the joy of laughter, the wonder of being alive.

Cobra: I shed the skin of this moment without fear, breathing into the next.

Corpse: Letting go, I release into the unknown.

Dancer: I dance to the song woven in my spine.

Downward Dog: May I become as authentic as a four-footed being.

Eagle: Seeing the world with clarity, I am poised to soar.

Fish: Through my throat, truth and light flow.

Forward Fold: Folding forward, I let go, letting my thoughts release.

Four-Limbed Staff: I hover, tapping into newly emerging strength.

Half-Fish: With confidence, I turn, diving deep.

Half-Moon: Suspended in space, I glow.

Headstand: Inverting, I open to a new point of view.

Knees-to-Chest: I embrace all that I am, all I have been, and all that I may become.

Legs-up-the-Wall: Becoming, temporarily, a corner—I pause.

Lion: Releasing all frustrations, I roar.

Locust: In the midst of swarming thoughts, I lift, becoming lighter with each breath.

Mountain: With stability, I weather all storms.

Plank: My arms, two pillars of strength, support me.

Plow: Overturning the soil, I ready myself for new growth.

Pyramid: Folding forward into the history and mystery of the practice, I breathe.

Reclining Twist: I breathe equally into my shadow and into my light, accepting both as part of me.

Seated Forward Fold: I bow to what is sacred in this life—from the children to the elders.

Seated Wide-Legged Forward Fold: I open authentically to my vulnerabilities, breathing in light.

Seated Twist: Turning to each side, I honor left and right, yes and no, end and begin.

Staff: Along the trellis of my upright spine, morning glories climb.

Tree: Rooting into my strength, I balance with ease.

Triangle: Accepting *was*, *is*, and *will be*, I integrate body, spirit, and mind.

Upward Dog: Heart shining, I face whatever comes, with love.

Warrior: Into conflict I gaze with courage, compassion, strength, and grace.

Wheel: I lift ever higher into the possibilities of this day.

ॐ Āsana Namaskāra

Oh, third limb of yoga, postures abounding,
you give us standing poses, seated poses,
twists, balancing poses, inversions...
You give us animals—Camel, Locust,
Downward Dog, Cat/Cow—
You give us shapes—Triangle, Bridge—
You give us Nature—Mountain, Tree, Half-Moon,
and positions beyond easy classification.
You, with your language of kinesthetic awareness
passed down through the ages,
our poses mirroring and echoing
the very stance of those who practiced generations ago,
they, with their own challenges and conflicts,
breathing deeply into their lungs, finding their balance,
equanimity, the same five elements—
ether, air, fire, water, earth—
nourishing them then as they nourish us now
as we take Child's Pose or *Chaturanga* or Cobra or Chair,
as we take *Garuḍāsana* or Gate,
Plank or Pyramid,
Knees-to-Chest or Legs-up-the-Wall,
Shoulderstand, Headstand, or Dancer,
we feel our muscles, we feel our bones,
we feel our breath,
we are alive,
we are present,
we are here.

Prāṇāyāma

The fourth limb of yoga, *Prāṇāyāma*, brings our attention to the breath.

ॐ The Life Force of *Prāṇa*

P*rāṇa* is the life force flowing through our bodies, our lives, our moment-to-moment interactions. Breathe. Feel the coolness of the air as it enters the twin portals of your nose on the inhale. Feel the warmth of the air as it exits the nostrils to join the atmosphere. Just as the invisible currents of Wi-Fi keep electronics connecting fluidly, the subtle *prāṇa*-carrying channels (*nāḍīs*) inside our body allow the various aspects of our psychophysiology to interconnect and flow. The circuitry of our nervous system, cardiovascular system, and respiratory system is charged by the current of *prāṇa*. Similarly, the life force of natural foods—foods that have not been frozen, microwaved, or otherwise distorted—is rich in *prāṇa*. We can go much longer without food, though, than we can without breath.

Prāṇa, when it is not obstructed through poor posture, unhealthy diet, or blockages at the physical, mental, and emotional levels, gives us a sense of ease. A sense of dis-ease intrudes when *prāṇa* is weak.

How many times do you check your phone each day? What if you were to check your breathing even half as often? Just as we may take care to charge our phone each day, we can charge our *prāṇa*. Sit quietly. For four minutes (or even two) watch your breath, listen to your breath, taste your breath, noticing how the texture of the breath feels as it travels through your nose, throat, and lungs, and then as it reverses the journey on the exhale.

ॐ Washing the Internal Pathways

We rejoice when a baby takes its first breath, and we watch closely as breath begins to exit the life of an elder. How often do we think of our breath, though, in all the years in between, in all the moments of our days? How often do we move beyond merely thinking about breathing and take action to do something to support our breath?

Prāṇāyāma, regulation of the breath, is an internal cleansing of the *nāḍīs* (subtle energy pathways). There are various forms of *prāṇāyāma*, and they can have a wide range of effects on the mind and body. For instance, a heating breath such as *Bhastrikā* (Bellows Breath) can remove stagnant air often associated with grief from the lungs, whereas a breath like *Bhrāmarī* (Bee's Breath) is soothing the nervous system, helping to calm anxiety and support sound sleep. (These breaths and others can be seen in the DVD *Pranayama for Self-Healing*, Lad 2009.)

If we're not used to taking time to work with the breath, the concept may seem a little strange. Breath is so constant in our lives that we can easily take it for granted; however, breath, as subtle as it is, is the determining factor between life and death.

When we stop and think about it, it is amazing that our breath continues, often for many decades, without any special care. Think about how often we defragment our computers, vacuum our homes, and get the oil changed in our cars. Can we similarly offer some loving maintenance and support of our breath, the one thing that separates us from death?

Note: *Prāṇāyāma* is a powerful practice with specific indications and contraindications, especially in regard to pregnancy and menses; it should be approached gradually and with the guidance of an experienced teacher.

ॐ Facets of the Prism

At first glance or thought, all breath is breath, just like snow seems like, well, *snow*, for one who only sees snow a few times a year or only during a few months of the year. It is when we become deeply familiar with something that we are able to notice and appreciate its nuances.

When we really look at snow, we may see snow sparkling in moonlight, snow glittering in sunlight, powdery snow, snow mixed with mud, snow glazed with ice, and so on.

Similarly, there are many different types of wind: Chinook, Santa Ana, Sirocco, White Squall, Westerlies, Polar Easterlies, trade winds, sea breezes, and many more.

As within, so without. In other words, our internal realms are, to a great extent, a microcosm of the natural environment. There is wind, for instance, in the body, Ayurvedically speaking, in the form of *Vāta doṣha*.

Therefore, when we pay attention, *really* pay attention, to the internal wind, or *prāṇa*, or breath in the body, we can notice differences— some subtle and some not so subtle at all. Of course we can notice hyperventilation, agonal breathing, the breath of a woman in labor, and other dramatic differences without much effort, but to tune into the day-to-day, hour-by-hour differences in our breath requires our attention.

Just as there are many types of winds, there are also many types of breath. For instance, within the realm of *prāṇāyāma*, there are very specific breaths that are quite different from one another: *Bhastrikā*, *Kapālabhāti*, *Anuloma Viloma*, and *Bhrāmarī*, just to name a few.

Even without moving into the intricate realms of *prāṇāyāma*, which are best studied with a teacher, we can notice aspects of our own breath. Is it slow? Is it fast? Is it shallow or deep? Where can you feel the breath in your body?

While we can approach this task of analyzing the breath as something to master, a test on which we wish to score 100 percent, this only takes us further into our mind, which can mean moving further away from the visceral experience of the breath.

Take some time right now and sit quietly. Without trying to change or fix your breath, just listen to it. Follow it. Feel it, noticing what you can observe in this moment.

ॐ Free

What in this life is free, truly free? Very little, it seems, and yet consider the fact that *prāṇāyāma* is available to us 24/7—and for no fee. The only cost, truly, is time, and the time commitment is quite minimal, unless many repetitions of many different *prāṇāyāmas* are being practiced. Is there any need for special equipment of any kind for *prāṇāyāma*? No. This means that *prāṇāyāma*, or the potential for it, is with us wherever we go, and we can tap into this wellspring of rejuvenation for no cost at all; it's free 365 days of the year.

Often, when something is advertised as "free," there is some gimmick. There is some fine print or there are some unseen strings attached. Therefore, we can shrink away from something that seems too good to be true.

With *prāṇāyāma*, the best way to determine if this deal is for real is simply to try it. Somewhere in the 1,440 minutes that you have each day, can you extract five minutes to give it a try, beginning with simply bringing your attention to the inhale and exhale? Would it be worth a five-minute daily investment to see what types of dividends you might receive?

Of course, dividends tend to accrue gradually, and the accumulated benefits may take some time to show. Then again, some *prāṇāyāmas* bring immediate effect, such as the energizing effect of *Kapālabhāti* (Skull-Shining Breath) or the calming effect of *Anuloma Viloma* (Alternate Nostril Breath). Ultimately, though, if we are attached to the idea of results, we may miss the process, so a certain amount of faith is needed.

Prāṇāyāma is a potent force. Tapping into this unsung hero of such a nourishing resource abiding within can change a life, not necessarily in a moment, or in a day, but breath by ever-unfolding breath.

ॐ Tempo, Texture, and Temperature

The sky is often just the sky, unless there is a dramatic sunrise or sunset. And unless giant storm clouds billowing in the distance catch our attention, we may just peripherally accept that a sky is there, without noticing if it is a royal blue sky, a pastel blue sky, a mottled sky, or an almost colorless sky. If someone were to ask you right now what today's sky is like, could you answer without going to the window?

We are often aware of so many things at once that our self-awareness falters. While we might juggle ten things in our mind at the same time, we may not know the rhythm of our own breath. We may not have any idea about the alignment of our spine. Although technically we are in our body, our mind may proceed like a remote operator rather than integrating with the body and soul to create a unified whole.

To explore the vast sea of the breath, we need only to become an open vessel, ready to observe. Look down at your body, at your abdomen, at your chest. What do you notice about the rise and fall of your breath? What is the tempo, the pace, the rhythm of your breath? Is it slow? Is it fast? Is it even or irregular? Does its tempo change as you bring your attention, your awareness to this motion?

Travel with the breath as it moves from the atmosphere into your nose and down your throat. What is its texture? Is it dry? rough? smooth? sharp? dull? Do you sense stagnation or an active, mobile quality? Perhaps there is an emotional texture to the breath as well. Is the breath light? heavy? Does the breath seem to hold sadness, worry, or joy?

As the air moves in through the nostrils, what is its temperature? Is it cool? Is it warm? Is it different on the inhale versus the exhale?

At times, when getting to know the breath, it can be helpful to assess the qualities of tempo, texture, and temperature. It is rather like assessing the basic qualities of an *āsana* when meeting it for the first time. Later, as time goes by, we can move past this basic assessment into the vast depths of experiencing the pose. Similarly, once we become comfortable staying with the breath, we can integrate our awareness with the breath itself by following the breath, letting it take the lead, being present for what unfolds.

ॐ Shared Thread

With the mind-boggling capacities of the internet, we are able to view the diversity of existence like never before. Not only are we able to see the incredible diversity of the human population from the Great Plains of the Dakotas and the mesas of the American Southwest to urban areas like New York, Paris, and Mumbai, we are also able to view the incredible array of species of four-leggeds, as well as winged and finned beings. The complexity of creation is, in many ways, beyond comprehension. And yet, there is a shared thread connecting all of us. This shared thread gently weaving us all together is the breath.

Breath courses through every single human being; humans of all ages, personalities, and careers breathe—criminals breathe, saints breathe, highly successful but possibly unhappy individuals breathe, the homeless breathe, children breathe, elders breathe, and everyone in between. We all breathe.

Recognizing this shared commonality offers a pathway into compassion. All of us have had those startling moments when we couldn't quite catch our breath due to overexertion, stress, shock, or some other factor. Similarly, we have all had at least one moment so wonderful that it nearly took our breath away. And regardless of the differing directions our lives have taken since birth, they all began in the exact same way: with breath.

The animal kingdom, too, from the gorillas and panthers roaming wild in the jungle to the beloved dogs and cats we call our pets to the whales and sharks swimming in the sea to the soaring ravens and hawks and crows and gulls and eagles above—they are all united by the shared thread of the breath.

Even cyberspace is strung with currents of *prāṇa*. As we consider the electronic energy that moves through online sites, fueling the search engine of our minds, we can counterbalance this by following the breath that powers the very vehicle that carries us, keeping us psychophysiologically balanced through the uploads and downloads of life.

ॐ *Prāṇāyāma Namaskāra*

Oh, *Bhastrikā, Kapālabhāti,*
Anuloma Viloma, Agni Sāra, Bhrāmarī,
Ujjāyi, Shītalī, Shītkāri, Udgīta,
more ways to taste the breath
than we can name or count,
infinite rhythms, textures, and speeds,
prāṇa, as gentle and as fierce
as the sky or sea,
as ancient and universal,
you
live within us
with your pulsing presence,
your life force measuring the length
of our lives, the ease or strain
of our days, and though we forget you
for hours or days at a time,
you carry on,
your devotion uninterrupted
day or night, keeping us afloat
in this life, able to receive
both the trials and treasures
of each new day

Pratyāhāra

....

Pratyāhāra, the fifth limb of yoga, relates to sensory perception, encouraging a withdrawal from excessive external stimuli.

ॐ A Center of Calm

Yoga studios are typically places of quiet. Sometimes gentle music is playing softly in the background. Imagine loud rock music pounding through the wall that a yoga studio shares with another business. This is a perfect opportunity to practice *pratyāhāra*, a pulling away from sensory stimuli or distractions. By choosing to turn the attention inward towards a center of calm (and away from the intrusive noise), the yogic limb of *pratyāhāra* is honored. A lot of energy could be expended being frustrated, disappointed, or angry, but if the loud music is accepted, attention falls away from it and towards the practice, deepening the practice at the physical level and beyond.

Throughout the day we have nearly endless opportunities to choose where we place our attention, our energy. Do notifications of each incoming message and update splinter our attention multiple times an hour, or do they reawaken our connectivity to others—or both? Observe your behavior during a typical hour. How many times do you check for texts, emails, social media posts, or other updates? What if you were to cut this number in half? What if you were to go thirty minutes or an hour without checking? Maybe it's not the phone—maybe it's the TV, radio, another electronic device, or a person drawing you in. Certainly there are countless benefits to the ways that communication enriches our lives on a daily basis. While we can love our electronic devices for the entertainment, information, education, and communication they make possible, being able to choose to use these devices with intention and for positive outcomes, rather than allowing them to swallow us, not only shifts our habitual patterns but also supports the calming of the nervous system. We can choose to pause, for instance, each time we hear or see a new message come in rather than immediately responding. Often we may not be able to perceive how "wired" we actually are until we offer *pratyāhāra* a chance to thrive.

ॐ Cellular Intelligence

With the great deal of importance that cell phones occupy in our society, they inevitably become part of the landscape of reality that shapes our lives. Recognizing the extensive powers of these devices, if we plug into the smartphone that resides within us, we may be surprised by our own capabilities. For example, in addition to using weather apps to monitor the temperature in external surroundings, we can periodically monitor the weather inside to see if we are feeling tired, anxious, excited, cloudy, stormy, sunny, clear, or something else.

There is also a lot of messaging or texting that takes place. Turning this communication flow inward, we can become receptive to messages from our internal environment. Check in with your ankles, knees, hips… your lungs, intestines, liver, throat, spine—how are they feeling? What are they messaging to you?

Similarly, GPS systems on phones guide us through the external terrain, helping us to arrive at locations we might not have found otherwise. With this inspiration, we can turn the attention inward, becoming more familiar with the internal terrain, observing areas of stiffness and ease, navigating to locate the origins of our grief and despair, the roots of our delight and peace.

Consider making the best of both worlds. For instance, each time your phone or computer makes a sound signaling a new message, welcome this as an opportunity to take a slow, deep breath. Let the notifications serve as awakenings, invitations to pause, rather than speed up. Just as incoming messages connect us to the outside world, they can also be gentle reminders to connect inside—with the emotions and with the breath.

You might also start seeing your phone as a way to find apps related to *āsana* and meditation, to sign up for yoga classes, to listen to calming music or chants, to view webcasts of yoga classes, meditation talks, yoga festivals, and spiritual teachings, or to program a daily reminder into your phone to power down, go within, and quietly observe the breath.

ॐ Powering Up by Powering Down

It can be surprising to notice how many things are powered up and running in our lives in any given moment. Look around. Are there lights on? How about heat or air conditioning or even a fan? Next, take inventory of electronic items that fall more easily into the optional category: TV, radio, computer, cell phone. Go further. Within that cell phone, how many apps are present, and how many are running? Are text messages coming in? Do alerts notify you each time an email comes in? What about the computer? How many different websites are up and running? These are some of the many things that may be going on when, in our drama-driven lives, we may feel that "everything's quiet" or even complain that "nothing's going on"; on the other hand, at other times, we may complain that we are overwhelmed and can't keep up with reading all the new posts/incoming messages and sending replies.

Is this something that the ancient sages had to contend with? While they were not walking around with smartphones tucked into their *sari* or *dhoti*, there was, as there has been in all culture and at all times, the challenge of external drama (events, gossip, social dynamics) and internal drama (emotions, thoughts, and conflicts between the two). *Pratyāhāra* guides us to be mindful of our interaction with these sources of stimulation or drama.

There are many ways we can support the process of *pratyāhāra*, which, in today's world, might be best understood as powering down. First, taking some time alone can help. This may mean going out into nature, such as a city park or even your own backyard, or it may simply mean choosing a room in your home where you can have some privacy. As we know, however, it's quite possible to be absolutely alone and still be "connected" to thousands if not millions of people through technology, or even connected to thousands of active thoughts, memories, and feelings even if we are not online. This is where the powering down comes in. Enter the stillness. Enter the quiet.

It's not uncommon, especially if you have a very high and sustained level of connectivity, to experience intense reactions, such as those that might accompany withdrawal from a drug habit, when powering down. If they come, observe them. Return to the breath. Follow the breath.

Stay within the breath as long as possible. If it helps to use a timer in the beginning, that's fine. Set it for five minutes and notice how long or short the five minutes feel. Increase the time span by a minute or more each day. In time, you will be able to enter into this space with less discomfort. In fact, there may come a time when you actually look forward to or even crave this quiet interlude in your day, and by taking mini-vacations from the electronic screens in your life, when you return to them it will be with renewed clarity and focus.

ॐ *Pratyāhāra* in the Midst

I n a time when many people are working more than one job; in a time
when credit card bills keep arriving; in a time when we are often
surrounded by others as we ride subways, buses, and other forms of
mass transit, it is often not possible to fit in a meditation retreat. It can
even be a major challenge just to "hide away" for ten minutes, depending
upon the living situation and the possible ongoing needs of children,
elders, spouses, pets, and so on.

What to do? Is it best to just throw our hands in the air and say,
"Well, it's just not possible for me to meditate"? While that may be an
understandable reaction, it may only further reinforce the belief of being
trapped, of being a victim to the complexity and intensity of the current
reality, whatever that may be.

Although it may seem unlikely, it's completely possible to withdraw
from the senses even in the midst of crowds and noise. Try this—either
literally or in your mind's eye: Sit in a crowded subway station on a bench.
Remove any headphones. Turn off your phone so that you are not hearing
any incoming texts or calls. Keeping your eyes open, turn the attention
inward. Even as you are aware of the people parading past you, you are
tuning into the realm inside. Where is your breath? Is it caught in your
throat? Is it stuck in the upper lungs? Does it seem to be roaming around
in your head? Breathe. Follow the breath, gradually slowing it down and
expanding it. Can you feel your feet? The soles of your feet? Your toes?
Your fingertips? Your core? The top of your head? Can you feel all of these
at the same time? Keep your eyes open. Breathe.

Working with being present in the world while also "tuning in" to
the Self is an ongoing practice that allows us to swim in the ocean of yoga
even when there is no possibility of getting to class or even to our mat. The
benefits of this training are immense, strengthening our concentration,
calming our nervous system, and allowing the brilliance of the braiding of
mind-body-soul to synchronize and sing.

ॐ Daily Dance

What is your daily dance? That is, on a regular basis, what is the choreography of your day? Is there a plan, a routine, or do you wake up and hope for the best? Hoping for the best, of course, can be a valuable approach in any situation, but the probability of a successful outcome is greatly enhanced by having at least one foot rooted in an intention or plan.

Āyurveda, the ancient sister science of yoga, recommends *dinacharyā*, which is a daily routine, to reduce stress and improve focus. By planning in advance what you will do upon waking, for instance, you take away the strain of needing to make that decision first thing in the morning, and by following a supportive routine, you can maximize your time. This, of course, is far from a militaristic schedule. Instead, it is a schedule that guides you to be able to have time and space for your priorities while maintaining a balanced lifestyle with adequate time for essentials, such as sleep.

How does this relate to *pratyāhāra*? When living in a society that pivots upon excitement, drama, and new information becoming available every moment, it is quite easy to become distracted. Having a daily plan can be a tremendously valuable buffer, allowing commitment to health and well-being to continue even in the midst of a busy life and unexpected events.

By choosing to move through life with *dinacharyā*, we support the idea of staying anchored amidst chaotic turns of events, integrating the daily responsibilities of work, family, and service to community with self-care. Part of this self-care is often a period of meditation, *prāṇāyāma*, and/or yoga *āsana*. Each time we take a step towards self-care and away from allowing ourselves to be swept away by tides that prioritize continual stimulation, whether in the form of electronics, caffeine, addiction to work, or something else, we give *pratyāhāra* a chance to breathe.

ॐ Extricating Ourselves

In ancient times, a web was the miraculously intricate symmetrical creation of an eight-legged being, and while these visual poems of gossamer still shine in the early morning dew from hidden corners outside from time to time, "the web" has taken on a completely different meaning.

The world wide web, a catalyst in connecting us with nearly all corners of the globe at all times, dazzles us with its ability to shrink limitations of time and space, and while the blessings of the convenience and information it delivers to us are many, it can also ensnare us, often without our awareness. Thread by thread, site by site, the web draws us in, absorbing inordinate amounts of our time, our attention, and sometimes even our money, if we let it.

For most of us, it would be undesirable or difficult, if not impossible, to abstain from using the internet. However, there are plenty of other webs that can entrap us. There are social dramas, of course, not to mention pledging our time and energy to various organizations. Commitments of any kind thread us together with others in ways that can support both ourselves and the community, but when the commitments overwhelm us and deplete us, they have become a web.

However, even if we abstain from social engagement and take time in solitude, we can still encounter webs that keep us from withdrawing our senses and embracing *pratyāhāra*. We can entertain and distract ourselves endlessly with the drama of our own mind. Memories, hopes, regrets, imaginations, worries, fears—there is endless material playing inside our minds, enough for many lifetimes of films. The movie is sometimes so vivid, so real, that it is easy to forget that it is the projection of our minds upon the screen of illusion. Choosing to turn off that movie, or at least place it on pause, can clear the path for *pratyāhāra*. This practice is so antithetical to much of modern society that it often needs beckoning, coaxing. Sitting in silence for five minutes each day is a sweet invitation to *pratyāhāra*. It says, "Welcome. I would love to get to know you better."

ॐ *Pratyāhāra Namaskāra*

Oh, wise one, beckoning us
inward when everything else
is calling to us like the Sirens' song
luring Odysseus from his path,
you offer us safe passage
into stillness, into quiet,
into turning notifications off,
TV off, DVD off, laptop off,
phone off, or turning them down—
not all the way or all the time,
but as needed, the oasis of calm inside
multiplying, flourishing,
able to soar in the deliciousness,
the spaciousness, the expansiveness
of being, integrated and centered,
the fragmented pieces defragmenting
as we power down, unplug,
power up the core,
plugging into the Self that, when extricated
from the hustle and bustle, can breathe,
recharging in a temporary fast
from the world of stimuli,
rejuvenating all of the five senses,
the entire system rebooting,
coming back online, refreshed.

Dhāraṇā

....

Dhāraṇā, the sixth limb of yoga, is concentration, the fixing of the mind on something internal or external.

ॐ Staying Centered

Dhāraṇā, one of the ancient limbs of yoga, continues to be vital today in our society that is nearly overrun by distractions. With incoming messages from all different directions all hours of day and night and with seemingly endless options of things to buy, places to go, shows to watch, and foods to eat, having the ability to focus can be an invaluable resource. At a time when so many children (and also adults) have been diagnosed with attention deficit disorder (ADD) and attention deficit hyperactivity disorder (ADHD), simply being able to concentrate can be a life-changing antidote for minds that constantly hop from one idea to another. However, *dhāraṇā*, concentration, is not as simple as it sounds. There are many ways that our own thoughts, as well as all of the distractions abounding around us, disrupt our concentration. Nevertheless, with dedication and practice, our capacity for concentration can flourish.

Try this: After you come home from your next yoga class, sit down and see how many of the poses you can list from recall; for a little more of a challenge, see if you can list the poses in the same order that you practiced them, perhaps even with details of the instructions.

ॐ Single-Pointed Attention

A re you a multi-tasker? There is sometimes a pride that enters into voices of people describing how they simultaneously tend to several different tasks at once, such as talking on the phone while checking their emails while cooking dinner. There is also sometimes a tension or despair in the same descriptions. Is it a victory to get three things done at a time instead of just one, especially when time is at such a premium that many people have turned to eating fast food or using microwaves to cook entire meals in minutes? What are the intangible costs of such speed? What does it mean when we no longer have time to sit quietly and read a book or have an uninterrupted conversation for more than five minutes?

The idea that "time is money" and "the more the better" can lead people to pile up three tasks at a time when years ago they would have had just one. This is like taking three plates instead of one when going through a buffet, and then trying to eat and digest all three plates of food at once.

We are often working so hard for so many hours and doing so many things at once that if we were to pause for just a moment, we might be quite challenged to remember the last fifteen minutes of what was said, done, and seen with much clarity. This is because when we enter into the realm of doing several things at once, quite a bit of dispersed mental activity is required, which is rather different from being present with the breath and concentrating on one thing at a time.

Ironically, it is sometimes possible to accomplish as much—if not more—when doing one thing at a time with complete focus as it is when doing multiple things at once. Try it for yourself for a few hours this week and see.

ॐ Mindfulness

When was the last time that you were present, fully present, as you ate? Eating is rarely a solo act. There is often reading, talking, walking, driving, watching TV, or something else involved in the process. Not only does this divert our mental attention, it also disperses our digestive fire, which may weaken our ability to absorb and assimilate nutrients.

What does food really taste like? Is it good? Delicious? Great! But what does it taste like? Is it salty? Sweet? Pungent? Astringent? Sour? Bitter? Is it some combination of these qualities? Are the foods crunchy? Dry? Smooth? Liquid? Oily? Do you eat them on autopilot, as quickly as possible, so that you can get back to what it was you were doing, or do you eat slowly, savoring each bite? Sometimes it is a particularly exquisite dessert that leads us to slow down and marvel, but what if we practiced this slow eating with awareness on a regular basis?

This type of slowing down can, ironically, actually speed up our progress on the way to *dhāraṇā*. Every daily contribution to this intention brings momentum. For instance, think about how often you walk during the day. It does not need to be a long walk on a beautiful trail. It can be the walk you take from your car to the grocery store, or your walk from your cubicle to the lunchroom. Mindfulness, a gentle awareness, can be brought with us as we walk. Paying attention to our breath, what we see, what we hear, what we smell, and what we feel as we walk can bring us into a place of real-time experience. This is quite different from the out-of-body experience of being a million miles away in our thoughts, and if this happens often enough, it may feel so familiar that we stop noticing the disconnect.

So whatever it is you choose to do this week, whether it is working in your garden, trading stocks, baking pies, sending emails, playing a sport, or something else, see how fully you can do it, bringing all of your capacities (seeing, hearing, tasting, smelling, touching) into focus. And if you notice that you are somehow proceeding as if by remote control, with your thoughts light years away from the task at hand, just notice. Sigh or laugh if you like. Return to your breath. Begin again.

ॐ A Mind Full of Fireflies

Have you ever seen fireflies light up a night sky, their pulsing lights blinking and moving through the dark? Sometimes our minds are like this, our thoughts zipping and flashing like lightning bugs late on a summer night. When ten or more thoughts are vying for our attention, we often begin trying to chase each one, tangling our mental focus and causing us to rush or become flustered, dissipating our energy.

Visualize the mind as this night sky full of fireflies, and then imagine these lights becoming the flame of a candle, a single focal point of attention. What is your chosen focus for this moment? If you like, you can choose to expand the time frame to encompass an hour, or longer.

It is difficult to be mindful when the mind is full of fireflies, yet when the mind is a single lit candle, the flow of attention has a focal point; thoughts and actions can align to that focus, delivering a sustained, rather than scattered, attention.

Sustainability of this mindset becomes possible with practice. So the next time your mind fills with fireflies, invite them to align, allowing a single flame of attention to shine.

ॐ Focus: Following the Gaze

Where are we looking? This is a question that can apply in an individual *āsana* and also throughout our daily lives, considering from moment to moment where our attention is focused.

When attention is keenly focused, it can have the power of a laser. When properly applied, as we know from medical technology, a laser can be lifesaving. When inappropriately applied, however, the laser-like attention can burn a hole right through a relationship or situation.

So where do you spend most of your time looking? Is it at screens? How often do your eyes move to your TV, your computer, and/or the small screen of your phone?

When you are walking, do you tend to look down, around, or up?

What about your internal gaze? Do you tend to look towards the past or the future? Does your gaze drift towards positive feelings and thoughts or towards the negative side of the spectrum?

What about in yoga class? Do you find yourself focused attentively on the *āsana* you are in, on the earrings dangling from the ears of the person in front of you, on the patterns of light coming through the window, or something else? Do you ever find your eyes drifting to the clock (if there is one) or to the thought of "how much longer?"—or are you so focused on what's going on that you are outside of time?

In yoga, the word *dṛṣhṭi* essentially refers to the gaze you might have in a pose. For instance, in Downward Dog, are you looking down at the ground, back at your feet, at your navel, or anywhere your eyes happen to land?

The next time you are lying on your back on your mat, become aware of your eyes. Are they moving upward towards the ceiling, or are they resting gently in your eye sockets? Are your eyes closed—and if so, are they focused on a particular *chakra* or another specific internal point, such as a muscle or organ, or are they roaming around in your to-do list, planning your next vacation, or something else?

Is it possible to keep your eyes open—aware and focused while simultaneously relaxed?

Change your gaze; change your life.

ॐ Of Pigeons and Pebbles

Your mind, filled with pebbles
and pigeons, squawking and feathers,
the uneven ground within you tumbling,
and you, sitting quietly,
counting your breaths,
losing count,
scolding or inviting yourself
to begin again,
the breath moving through you,
finding your stiff places,
your stuck places,
the knotted spaces untangling
in the language of spheres
moving beyond logic
and you, looking the same
from the outside,
your mind quiet now, and still,
even if just for this moment,
the peacefulness of a starry sky
where pigeons once stumbled and squawked.

ॐ The Energy of Attention

What did you do yesterday? Were you on autopilot going through the same schedule that you follow on a regular basis, or did you move through this familiar schedule with awareness? Did you drift through the day letting one thing evolve into the next? While there are many ways to move through the day, the accumulation of choices we make in each moment ultimately creates the fabric of our lives.

Setting an intention is one way to spark awareness and direct the gaze of our lives. This does not need to be a formal setting of intention; it can happen in a brief moment upon waking, or in a moment before getting out of the car to head into the office.

Your intention may be something very specific, such as "I will respond to the eight emails that are most pressing before lunch," or they can be more comprehensive, such as "I will pause each time before I speak or write, responding with compassion each time."

When we have an intention as a target or guide, it directs our energy and efforts, much in the same way that a flame of a candle draws in our attention in the practice of *trāṭaka*.

To practice *trāṭaka*, sit quietly in front of a candle for several minutes. Keep your gaze soft and fixed on the candle's flame. Afterwards, you might take a few moments to journal your experience, considering how you might bring a similar focus to a situation in your life.

Ultimately, where attention goes, *prāṇa* (our breath, our life force) flows. What are the top three things you could focus on that would serve your life, and the benefit of the community, the most?

Such an internal gaze can be subtle and easy to lose track of. Checking in at the end of each day, week, and month can be a healthy way to assess how reality is correlating with your intention in terms of where your focus is going. Allow the focus to change, as needed, as the weeks continue. Impermanence is an unavoidable part of this life, and being responsive to the shifting tides of life can keep our gaze authentic, serving our lives and the lives of those around us with grace.

ॐ Awareness without Anticipation

O
ften in this life we are already thinking about the next thing we want to accomplish before even completing the current task at hand. How many times have you anticipated the cue of a yoga teacher whose style you are familiar with, moving your body before the words of instruction came? Although being able to move in a familiar flow can be helpful, this type of autopilot *āsana* practice short-circuits the opportunity to pause, knocking our gaze or attention out of alignment with the present state of our body and being.

This may often happen seemingly on its own. We may find ourselves mentally drafting a letter during Bridge Pose or planning out our next day as we drive home from work. In some regards, this approach may be born from not wanting to be caught off-guard, unprepared. However, when we let go into the moment, our mind, body, and breath begin to synchronize. Depending upon the actual situation, this can make the moment more or less difficult. For instance, we might just feel a long-ago grief (that we thought was healed) well up as a hip opens if we are not busy distracting ourselves with thoughts of could be, would be, should be. When we stay with what is, at first quite a bit of discomfort, unease, and even fear can arise, usually in proportion to how strongly we've blocked these feelings. Tears may come; there may be shaking. This is all good evidence that what has been stagnant is unlocking. Eventually, if we stay with this process, accepting it gently, there can be a softening as the body, mind, and spirit begin to work harmoniously.

When the dissonance of cacophony shifts into a greater sense of harmony, this internal balancing will support the ability to enter more fully into *dhāraṇā*. When the mind is no longer fighting and has given up its habitual patterns, it begins to open to feeling the full gamut of physical sensations that may be present, as well as emotions that may be there. The flow of attention can then become less obstructed; concentration can improve.

The next time you finish a pose, see if you can come out of it with as much attention as you went into it. In the same way that we often pop out of a pose, we often pop out of one experience, thought, or emotion and into another, and while this type of speedy transition can be important in an emergency, let's hope that each moment of our life is not an emergency. By training our brain to engage with the body in yoga *āsana*, through the generous thread of the breath, we can, in time, transition more gracefully in our day-to-day happenings when we are off the mat. Try it right now. What is your next step? Connect in with the breath first, and then proceed, keeping the attention flowing, moving slowly, with awareness, into that next step.

ॐ Attention and *Māyā*

R eading and thinking about concepts, such as *dhāraṇā* and the other seven limbs of yoga, is all well and good; however, it is not a substitute for the actual experience of these concepts. We can read and write about these topics, and listen to lectures about these concepts, but that does not necessarily mean that we are any closer to actually integrating them into our lives. Distinguishing between guides to our practice and the practice itself is important. We can easily fan the flame of the ego by thinking that we are knowledgeable about yogic philosophy, yet notice how much more challenging it is to practice even one part of one yogic limb, such as contentment (*santoṣha*), than it is to talk for hours about all eight yogic limbs.

After all, where is the value in practicing *āsana* for an hour, and then going out into the world and reverting to habits that fall outside of yogic ideals?

Keeping our attention and concentration on reality will ultimately serve us much better than being swept away by the *māyā*, or illusion, that we are somehow more advanced simply because we are reading, writing, or thinking about *dhāraṇā*, or any of the other limbs of yoga.

ॐ *Dhāraṇā Namaskāra*

Point of focus, you draw us in,
and as you draw us in,
we let go, inch by inch,
millimeter by millimeter,
of all that vies for our attention,
disentangling our thoughts and habits
from all that seeks to take us
away from our focus.

Thank you for receiving us,
for receiving the attention
of our eyes, our minds,
our hearts, for being
the process through which we find
ourselves, even as we find you,
as we slip away,
distracted again,
only to return,
to renew
our concentration,
humbled again
by the challenge
of holding our attention
in one single place.

Dhyāna

....

The meditative state of *dhyāna*, the seventh limb, may emerge over time from a sustained practice of *dhāraṇā*.

ॐ Suspended in Time

Over time, the one-pointed concentration of *dhāraṇā* may become the more spacious, flowing meditative state of *dhyāna*. In our world of traffic and forty-hour (or longer) workweeks, however, where is the time and space for sustained meditation? Is it enough to know that deep in the Himalayas there are yogis sitting in caves in meditation for hours and days and weeks on end, or do we wish to meditate, too? With awareness of how fully scheduled many lives are, how might we sample at least a taste of the banquet of benefits that meditation serves?

In our point-and-click modern culture, we become accustomed to speedy service and lightning-fast results. Waiting on hold for a full two minutes on the phone can elicit a volcano of frustration and aggravation. In many places, the world has become a culture of action and speed. Where, then, is the respect for sitting motionless without anything tangible to show for the time? In a culture that often equates time with money, recognizing the intangible benefits of meditation necessitates a shift in awareness.

Those unable to accept the words of sages or to simply have faith in the experiences of those who have devoted much of their lives to meditation may find it useful to review scientific studies on the benefits of meditating. Often, the most convincing path, however, is simply to experience meditation and see what is felt and observed. There may be some discomfort physically, mentally, and emotionally at the outset, but over time, like a pathway being cleared of debris accumulated from many years, a sense of ease can come.

ॐ Mini-Meditations

Sometimes people decide that they are going to meditate and just dive in, pushing themselves to begin with sitting in meditation for fifteen or thirty minutes. While this is definitely a reasonable period of time for an experienced meditator, sitting for this amount of time as a newcomer can overload the system. In the beginning period of a meditation practice, as the debris of the mind begins to come up for review before being washed clean, there may be a mixture of thoughts, memories, and emotions. This period may feel unsettling rather than the calm typically associated with meditation, and the support of a meditation teacher can be invaluable.

It can also help to start small. Planting seeds of meditation in increments of even a few minutes of stillness at a time can grow into a steady and fulfilling meditation practice that will shelter like the grace of a forest that has been rooted in the earth for many, many years.

Once the mind begins to empty into the still waters of peace, it will be able to return to this state more easily. Considering how many thousands of thoughts speed through our neural pathways on a regular basis, it makes sense that slowing these runaway trains of thought takes some time. The mind, like a wild animal, may resist training at first. Patience is vital during this process as well as a gentle acceptance that each session will be different. Welcoming the journey and its full range of unexpected destinations (even while sitting still) can open the mind and heart, inviting old patterns that are no longer needed to release and let go.

Sit quietly. Breathe. Observe. Notice any judgments and return to the breath. Allow yourself to feel the spaciousness beginning to unfold.

ॐ Early Morning

There is a beautiful stillness in the early hours of morning. The mind, still steeped in ambrosia of sleep, has not yet jumped into its racing patterns of mental activity. It has not yet been stimulated by caffeine, noise, the glare of computer screens, or the digestion of food. In this sacred time of transition between the deep leagues of sleep and the active pace of daylight hours, the mind can be nourished by rooting into a stillness, into quiet.

Truly, meditation can take place anytime and anywhere, and a very experienced meditator could drop into stillness in the midst of a loud crowd, but the early morning hours are especially ripe for entrance into meditation. Through this portal of dawn, we can enter into the cosmos of peace.

There is also a cosmos within—the cosmos of the stars and galaxies of our minds and hearts, the planets of our soul. In meditation, we have the capacity to tap into this vast realm in a wordless way, freeing the mind from its typical role of thinking. Simultaneously, we are part of the external cosmos, from the etheric level of the galaxies above to the realms of earth, water, fire, and air.

Imagine how the world might hum if even 50 percent of the population awoke and sat in meditation for five minutes.

ॐ Continuous Flow

S wimming a lap across the pool requires enough stamina to enter into a flow. Whether it is freestyle or backstroke, the arms and legs propel the body in a continuous flow from one edge of the pool to the other. Given the tremendous concentration and effort this takes, the swimmer may pause before pushing off for the next lap. However, after a certain length of time and regular practice, the swimmer will be able to swim many laps without stopping. When this repetitive motion is sustained without overexertion, a deeper sense of flow can occur as the swimmer glides back and forth across the pool maybe twenty times or more.

Similarly, when we become practiced enough in *dhāraṇā* (concentration), we may, at some point, enter into *dhyāna*, a continuous flow of meditation. For instance, if your object of concentration is a word, you might return to this word many times throughout the day and eventually throughout each hour, but when you live this word, breathe this word, and this word comes to live in your consciousness continuously, this is the realm of *dhyāna*.

ॐ Deeply Immersed

B ecoming deeply immersed is a way to have a taste of what it might feel like to be able to sit completely still and have the mind so relaxed, so content that everything else falls away. While this level of flow may sound impossible or unattainable in this lifetime, consider this—have you ever had hours fly by when you were focused on something, such as playing a sport, creating artwork, cooking, or gardening? If so, you have tasted *dhyāna*.

Remember when you first learned to drive? Likely you took short practice drives, and the small acts of starting, stopping, accelerating, and braking took a great deal of concentration. Now, almost without thinking, you could probably drive for hours, or as far as your fuel tank could take you, in a continuous flow.

The journey can seem impossible when we look at a map, but when we allow ourselves to begin, we put ourselves in the position for change to occur as we travel into the unknown, with awareness of the many others who have followed this path before us.

ॐ *Dhyāna Namaskāra*

Continuously flowing, like the sea,
you do not stop, and we,
challenged by our stop-and-go
point-and-click lives,
don't always flow with you,
and yet you wait, never flinching,
never despairing, always available,
never turning us away
for failed attempts
no matter how long or how far we've been away,
inviting us to experience
even if only for just a few moments,
a continuous flow
a sustained concentration
an uninterrupted focus
a perpetual awareness
of being,
undiluted, unpolluted
by distraction
or contraction
of mind or breath
flowing deeply
flowing smoothly
resonating
with the full embodiment
of every molecule,
every breath.

Samādhi

....

Samādhi is the eighth limb of yoga.

ॐ Going Beyond

How do we hold the concept of *samādhi* in our minds? Is it not like imagining a country we have never visited? Today we have endless photos and videos of most places available online, reducing the mystery of a faraway place, yet not too long ago these places resided in the vast realms of imagination except for those whose feet had walked the soil, whose eyes had seen the flora and fauna, whose mouths had tasted the cultural delicacies specific to the region, whose noses had smelled the scents of these foods and the aromas of the local flowers, and whose ears had heard the melodies of the bird calls and cadences of the foreign languages.

Similarly, only those sages and enlightened beings who have experienced *samādhi* truly have a sense of this eighth limb of yoga—and it may be, in many ways, ineffable. While the experience may move beyond the realm of communication, we can perhaps have a taste of what *samādhi* may be like when we enter so fully into an experience that we lose the limitation of time and space, moving into a space even deeper than *dhyāna*. In such a profound state, we may experience the bliss of being unified within ourselves and with the cosmos, while simultaneously being freed from the confines of any limitations.

ॐ Bliss

When was the last time you felt the deep sense of contentment and joy that comes from being aligned with a genuine sense of purpose or an intangible experience of pleasure? How often do you feel nourished by a healthy activity, such as painting, hiking, gardening, playing music, or visiting with a friend? These are moments that draw us closer to the delicious realm of bliss.

What is bliss? Is it a sense of awe we feel when the stars in the night sky over the open prairie are so bright that we forget our worries and pain? Is it the sweet peace of floating on a raft feeling the gentle undulation of the waves beneath and the warmth of a sea breeze all around? Moments like these take us outside of ourselves, reducing our concerns, frustrations, and grief while giving us a more joyous perspective within the context of the cosmos.

Even a second when the mind stills is like a pocket of light in the midst of a clouded sky. It may not be much, but it points to an expanse of light and calm that exists and may become accessible at any moment.

ॐ How Long Will It Take to Get There?

O ften a young child who is on a long trip will repeatedly ask, "How much longer?" and while this repeated question can become comical or even frustrating as the hours roll by, is this really much different than what can take place in the adult mind as it becomes impatient with progress toward a goal? While having a goal or destination in mind can bring a sense of purpose, direction, and motivation, focusing too much on a goal can rob us of what is right in front of us. Does the impatient child on a long trip notice the charming dog in the car that just zipped by or the unusual shape of the cloud that just passed outside the plane window?

Like this child fixated on the unseen destination, we, too, can miss what's in our midst. When the focus on getting to the next step on the path becomes too strong, then the mind is anticipating the next moment rather than experiencing the current one. Rather than looking to the next class, pose, or a further perfection of a familiar pose, or reaching for a deeper level of concentration or meditation, we can listen to the inhale and exhale of the breath, noticing the waves of thought in our mind.

Samādhi, like grace, will arrive when and if it arrives, not a moment too soon or a moment too late, but if we're always trying to race ahead of where we are, we just might miss it—and a lot of other beautiful things along the way. It's like trying to get to another country without a passport or trying to access a secure website without a password. When we can accept where we are, and appreciate it, both its challenges and its gifts as part of the journey, perhaps that in itself is a tiny taste of the sweetness of *samādhi*.

ॐ What Is?

I n this age when libraries and bookstores are filled with books and even more information is available online, there can be a belief that if something is real, if it exists and is knowable, then it can be read about. Is this so? For those who believe truth is always quantifiable through scientific data and qualifiable through description, reality is tangible.

For others who may have experienced something that could not easily be measured or fit into language, they may have a different perspective. For instance, there can be many paradoxes in yoga, such as being in a relaxed state with full awareness, or aiming for progress along the path without having any attachment to that goal.

Samādhi rests as the deep eighth level in the ocean of yoga. Just as only the most experienced of deep-sea divers would even think of going to the bottom of the sea, *samādhi* may, in this lifetime, be out of reach. However, just knowing that such a peaceful, blissful state exists can support us when we feel mired in day-to-day responsibilities.

Even within *samādhi*, there are multiple layers or levels, the ocean of yoga ever replete with mystery. Accepting that *samādhi* is a place we may or may not ever visit, what can we do today to bring forth more peace and bliss into our life or the life of another?

ॐ Deep Peace

Deep peace
born of millennia
of ebb and flow,
celestial music
moving through the veins,
the stars speaking
a language beyond grammar,
past, present, future
folding into themselves
like a fragrance
waking memory and dream
in the same breath,
the battle between
action and stillness
converting to dust,
ocean waves turning
shells from sand,
candlelight blooming,
repeated prayers,
the *mantra* beyond *mantra*
charging the lungs with new wings,
syllables rich as the finest silks,
the heart like a cathedral
rose window, sunlight streaming in

ॐ *Samādhi Namaskāra*

Union, bliss, peace,
our words faltering
as we approach you,
the realms of your grace
mystifying our minds
built as they are on logic,
infused as they are
with doubt and fear.
You, shining in the distance,
are beyond our beyond,
our ability to receive you
dwarfed by the mountains
we have not yet climbed,
or seen.

You, though you have been
written about, read about,
wondered about, and talked about,
reside far beyond all this,
just as the music of the moon's luminosity
dwells far beyond the reaches of sound.

Thank you, liberating essence,
illimitable,
residing in a dimension
science may never know,
you,
the sweetest of nectars,
you
the Divine's
exquisite glow.

ॐ How Many Limbs?

In a yoga *āsana* practice, we are sometimes on four limbs, such as in Plank, *Chaturaṅga*, Downward Dog, or Wheel. Other times we are on two limbs, such as Triangle, Half-Moon, or Chair. Still other times, we balance on one limb, like in Eagle or Tree or Warrior 3. In all of these poses, we are within the third limb of yoga—*āsana*.

How many of the eight limbs of yoga can we practice at the same time? If we are in a pose, such as Chair, in addition to *āsana*, we can integrate a *yama*, such as *ahiṃsā* (non-violence, doing the pose safely and compassionately). We might also bring to mind a *niyama*, such as *tapas* (burning impurities through disciplined practice) or *santoṣha* (being content with our current pose).

Additionally, we can take our attention to the breath (*prāṇāyāma*), focusing on a slow, deep, even breath. We might also take our gaze to a specific point in front of us, practicing concentration (*dhāraṇā*). We may even enter a pose so deeply that, as we hold the pose, our concentration becomes meditation (*dhyāna*).

If these multiple limbs of yoga can join together in *āsana*, can they not also join together in other moments of our life?

For instance, imagine you're in a restaurant and you're waiting for your order for an unusually long amount of time. Will you practice *satya* (truth) in notifying the wait staff of how long you've been waiting? Will you practice *aparigraha* (non-grasping) and relax your grip on needing to be served quickly? Will you practice *svādhyāya* (self-study), reflecting on how pleasantly or unpleasantly you have been communicating (or thinking) about the situation? Will you check your posture (*āsana*)? Will you pay attention to your breath (*prāṇāyāma*)? Will you take the opportunity of this extra time to focus (*dhāraṇā*) on something positive, such as the person sitting across from you? Is it possible you might even enter into a brief meditation (*dhyāna*) as you wait?

Like an internal compass of eight directions—north, south, east, west, northeast, northwest, southeast, southwest—the eight limbs of yoga exist as they have for ages, as relevant to the mapping of our lives today as they have been for generations.

ॐ Applying the Eight Limbs

I t's one thing to study the eight limbs of yoga. It's another thing entirely to try to integrate them into our practice on the mat and in our lives.

It can be a feat to simply memorize the list of *yamas* and *niyamas*. To practice, recall a recent situation you have experienced. Then, see how many ways you can relate each of these ten facets of the first two limbs of yoga listed below to the situation:

- *ahiṃsā* (non-violence/compassion)

- *satya* (truth)

- *asteya* (non-stealing)

- *brahmacharya* (conservation of vital energy)

- *aparigraha* (non-grasping)

- *shaucha* (cleanliness, purification)

- *santoṣha* (contentment, acceptance)

- *tapas* (self-discipline)

- *svādhyāya* (self-study, reflection)

- *Īshvara praṇidhāna* (surrendering, faith in the divine).

Five Obstacles: *Kleshas*

In Sūtra 2.3 of Patañjali's *Yoga Sūtras*, he states the five *kleshas*: *avidyā*, *asmitā*, *rāga*, *dveṣha*, and *abhinivesha*. *Kleshas* are essentially obstacles along our yogic path.

ॐ Obstacles Along the Path

Have you ever been driving and had an 18-wheeler truck pull out in front of you, obscuring your view of what was ahead? Have you ever had these trucks also appear in the lanes to your left and right, boxing you in? These are challenges in the journey, just like the debris that sometimes will land on the road right in front of us with little or no time or space for us to swerve to avoid it. Just as there are physical obstacles or challenges along the roads we travel in the world, so too are there internal obstacles on our path. These are described in the *Yoga Sūtras* as afflictions, or *kleshas*.

ॐ A Little Ignorance Goes a Long Way (*Avidyā*)

I gnorance (*avidyā*) is known as the primary *klesha* (affliction), leading to the other four afflictions, which, like ignorance, can cause suffering. We can think of ignorance as a lack of information in the form of data. For instance, someone who is not on social media may not be aware of certain happenings, and those who do not tune into news on the television, radio, or internet may be uninformed about specific events taking place in the local, national, or global community. However, ignorance in the classical sense extends far beyond this type of lack of data.

We can have all of the most current data at our fingertips and still be ignorant. We might be unaware, for instance, of how these pieces of information relate to each other or the deeper meaning of this data. In other words, we might have the knowledge of a situation but not have wisdom about its full significance. Furthermore, we may be ignorant about the events inside our own selves. These events may be thoughts, emotions, memories, or ideas. We may be so bombarded by information and events from the outside world that we are not tuned into the events and information unfolding within, or vice versa. We may also not have a pathway to process the type or amount of information—whether internal, external, or combined—in a meaningful or healthy way. All of these scenarios, and others, can lead to ignorance.

What can we do? Are we doomed to ignorance? While there is always the potential for clouds of ignorance to move in and cover the light of awareness, by taking silence to pause and observe, pause and reflect, pause and digest, we reduce the potential for our minds and hearts to be compromised by a build-up of the sludge that can form when we are racing from one thought to another, one activity to another. *Āsana* practice, meditation practice, and *prāṇāyāma* practice are all helpful ways to slow down and offer awareness the chance to strengthen and become more present in our daily lives.

ॐ Meek or Overly Confident or Somewhere in Between (*Asmitā*)

smitā refers to ego-related afflictions (*kleshas*). If the ego is inflated, there can be a sense of being better than others, which can lead an individual to become conceited or vain. This over-exaggerated sense of importance can cause a person to have an aggravated sense of ambition and to treat others with a lack of respect.

In contrast, if the sense of the ego is deflated, a person may feel very unsure of his or her value or importance in this life. The insecurity, low self-esteem, and self-doubt can combine to make the person fearful, depressed, or even despondent.

Clearly, neither one of these extremes of ego is ideal, and while we may vacillate from time to time between feeling more important or less important than we actually are, the more we can stay in touch with an accurate sense of who we are and our worth as a human being, the better chance we have of moving through life with the support of an authentic center. When we find the middle ground, genuinely acknowledging our own worth as well as the worth of others, we move towards equanimity.

Sometimes the things that skew our sense of self and our place in the world are quite basic. For instance, when we are overtired, we may not process thoughts and emotions in the way that we might if we were more fully rested. We may also not be at our best if we are not eating nutritiously and receiving proper nourishment.

Nourishment comes in many forms. For instance, even if we are eating a well-balanced diet but do not have companionship, our loneliness and sense of isolation may affect our digestion and make issues that might ordinarily feel quite manageable seem insurmountable. When our minds are overworked or aggravated by criticism or negative influences, the balance of our thinking will be affected.

Therefore, the more we can have a balance of work and rest, as well as solitude and togetherness, the better able we are to keep our mind, body, and spirit in a place of health, allowing our ego to stay in check.

ॐ Pulled Like a Magnet (*Rāga*)

A ttachment (*rāga*) is an affliction in which we bind ourselves to previous experiences in a way that makes us crave more of the same. It is only natural to hope for positive experiences, but expecting or needing to feel the same pleasure as we did yesterday or last week or last year limits us by blocking us from experiencing the present moment.

For example, if you happened to see the sunset yesterday and it was gorgeous, and if you see the sunset today and it does not look the same, you may be disappointed rather than open to receiving the beauty of the unique way the sun has chosen to depart from daylight today. In truth, each sunset is absolutely beautiful if we open our minds and hearts to the new experiences each day has to offer.

Similarly, if we are overly attached to a certain person or even the behavior or words of that person on a certain day, then we deny ourselves the opportunity to embrace the full nature of the person and humanity as a whole. Each of us is changing on a daily basis; even hour to hour we may be different in terms of our moods, our energy levels, and the clarity of our thinking and our communication. Allowing our expectation for things to remain as they were in the past (whether that past is an hour ago, a day ago, or a year ago) to shift to a more spacious acceptance of the fluctuations of life can reduce our suffering by replacing our longing and disappointment with a curiosity about what may unfold in the next moment, the next hour, the next day, and the next week. This can be therapeutic as long as we do not then become attached to expectations for the future.

Think about what you have your heart set on doing later today or later this week. Measure your attachment to this plan on a scale of 1 to 10. See what it takes to loosen this hold, this grip you have on wanting or needing the plan to work out. It's not that we stop caring or hoping for a favorable outcome; it's a matter of opening ourselves to the reality that in the complex configuration of life, things may change between now and then. It's allowing the awareness of our small place in the vast universe to bloom and nourish us as we journey, breath by breath, into the unknown.

ॐ Recoiling (*Dveṣha*)

I s there a city or country that you have wanted to visit for many years? Is there a food that you absolutely adore? Just as we can feel strongly attracted to specific places, people, and experiences, we can also have aversion to certain people, places, and situations. This type of repulsion is known as *dveṣha*. While becoming unduly attached to anything can bring its own flock of miseries, going out of our way to avoid certain things is also a behavior linking us to suffering.

Why do we avoid a certain person or situation, for instance? Often, it is because we remember a previous experience with this person or situation that was unpleasant. It might even be that a certain person or experience simply reminds us of someone or something similar that was unpleasant. Naturally, we do not wish to be drawn back into an emotional vortex of fear, anger, grief or other difficult feelings, so we may make excuses (consciously or subconsciously) to try to protect ourselves. However, by doing so, we are, in a sense, allowing the past to control us. By clinging to a belief that events and feelings will unfold in the exact same way that they did before, we may be clinging to fear and also a possible need for control.

Certainly, we do not need to put ourselves unnecessarily into the path of emotional pain or discomfort; however, by loosening our grip on the past and on our fears, we can enter into each interaction and inner conversation fresh with the possibility for it to be one of renewal rather than one doomed to repeat difficulties of the past.

This is easier said than done; however, disciplining ourselves to practice at least one of the limbs of yoga on a regular basis (daily, if possible) can help to remove or reduce mental, emotional, and physical blocks by cleansing the subtle internal energetic pathways (*nāḍīs*).

It may even be a yoga pose or type of yoga pose that we resist. Opening the mind and heart to this awareness can be the beginning of transformation.

Even if it's not possible to do a full *āsana*, *prāṇāyāma*, or meditation practice each day, do a little. The little can grow over time, but for now, the little is a lot—much more than none at all.

ॐ Hanging on for Dear Life (*Abhinivesha*)

Are you ready to die? Does this question bring a resounding "no" or a jolt of fear? When we examine our thoughts and feelings around one of the only guaranteed experiences of this life—death—a wide variety of responses can emerge in varying degrees of intensity. When we have significant aversion to the thought of dying, this is a form of *abhinivesha*, or clinging to life, which is the fifth *klesha* or affliction.

Clinging to life, to a certain degree, is necessary and useful; however, when our aversion to death is so strong that it begins interfering with our ability to live in the present moment, we have entered into unnecessary suffering.

Death, a change of forms, often brings to mind the moment when *prāṇa*, or life force, exits the body, and yet death is present in many forms and occurring on a daily, hourly basis. Plans are dying, relationships are dying, businesses are dying, traditions are dying, and while all of this may sound rather depressing, these deaths allow births to take place in the rhythmic cycle of give and take.

While the metaphorical death of a relationship or job can feel devastating, many times these dramatic shifts clear space and energy for a new path that may ultimately be equally or even more fulfilling, even though this may seem impossible at the time.

Therefore, by clinging to the way things are and insisting that they do not change at all, we block the natural flow of life, which can lead not only to stagnation emotionally and mentally, but also physically.

As with most aspects of this life, when we can find a balance, we thrive. If we can embrace life with nutrition, nourishment, moderate exercise, adequate rest, joy, and forgiveness without clinging to life and without having undue fear of death, then we become vessels for transformation, allowing us to minimize our suffering and maximize the ways in which we can be a light to ourselves, to our families, our friends, our communities, and the world.

It begins with the breath. If we can follow our breath, without holding our breath or forcing our breath, we can stay present. As long as we are present, we are alive and moving in a direction that will ease our transition into death whenever it may come, whether that may be tomorrow, next week, next year, or ten, twenty, thirty, forty, fifty, sixty, seventy, or eighty years from now.

ॐ *Klesha Namaskāra*

You, ancient stumbling blocks
tripping us still,
you, like the stern teacher
who keeps holding a mirror
to us, showing us
ourselves,
you appear and disappear,
reappearing just when we think
we have moved past you,
our ignorance,
our attachments,
our aversions,
our distortions of self,
our fears of death
all alive and well,
perhaps weaker or stronger
depending upon the day,
the gifts of your obstacles
shaping us, humbling us,
bringing us to our knees
as we return, stumbling, crawling
to practice, beginning anew.

Seven Spinning Wheels: *Chakras*

ॐ Circles of Light

There are many different understandings of *chakras* and while the rich intricacies of *chakras* are likely only accessible by advanced Sanskrit scholars, *rishis*, sages, and *sādhus*, we can have, with awareness, appreciation for the subtle realms of our anatomy. One understanding of *chakras* is that they are circles of light, spinning wheels, or energetic centers within. In these seven centers dwell mysteries untold, unfolding with each breath. Do we see them? Feel them? Placing our hands on the seven *chakras* brings the esoteric and the tangible together, gently. Each of these seven centers has a story to tell. Like the seven continents forming the landscape of our globe, they help shape the world within.

ॐ Rooting into Life: *Mūlādhāra Chakra*

Hidden beneath the magnificence of any tree is a vast realm of support. The roots sometimes travel for many feet, seeking the nourishment the tree requires. The support from below allows the trunk to stand firmly and the branches to expand, mirroring the parallel expansion of the roots underground.

Like a tree, we, too, have our roots, and though they are not visibly attached to us in ever-lengthening tentacles, they serve us in similar fashion, supplying us with nourishment.

What is at the root of your life? Is it your career? A relationship? An ambition? An addiction? A regret? A hope? Something else? On a scale of 1 to 10, how supported do you feel in your life? Who in your life accepts and appreciates you just as you are, knowing the full range of your qualities?

In what ways do you provide a foundation of support for yourself? A regular practice of meditation, *prāṇāyāma*, *āsana*, journaling, prayer, or self-reflection can provide nourishment—mind, body, and soul—that can offer tremendous support to *mūlādhāra*, the root *chakra*, which, in turn, supports our overall well-being. Our basic survival issues, such as safety and security, manifest here with the boldness of the red color, the right to be alive.

While there are various *mantras* and *āsanas* said to support each *chakra*, perhaps the first step is to examine life with honest, loving eyes to understand:

- What would your being benefit from rooting into more? (This might be a type of food, a daily practice, balanced finances, a type of relationship, nature, rest, etc.)

- What would your being benefit from rooting into less? (This could be processed or microwaved food, excessive use of electronics, gossip, self-judgment, overworking, suppressing emotions, overspending, etc.)

If the health and stability of our *mūlādhāra chakra* directly corresponds to the choices we make regarding what we root into, moment by moment, what do you choose to root into today? What do you choose to root into now?

ॐ Creating Anew:
Svādhiṣṭhāna Chakra

Creativity is the wellspring of our life force. After all, without the creative force of procreation, our individual life would not have come into being. And yet, creativity exists far beyond the realm of procreation. Every word we speak, every thought we think, every action we take is, at its root, a creative force. However, many people will claim they are not creative. Not everyone can find a solution to a complex mathematical equation or paint a portrait or design a new app, but we all embrace creativity each day that we are alive as we interact with and respond to the dynamic environment of life around us.

The second *chakra*, *svādhiṣṭhāna*, relates directly to creative flow through its association with the water element. Sometimes we feel we are "in the flow," where life is unfolding fluidly and we are moving along with few obstacles or interference. This is the wealth of a healthy *svādhiṣṭhāna*. Our capacity to bring forth newness, whether that is a baby, a song, a video, a recipe, a garden, an architectural design, or something else, is boundless. Looking at how we honor creativity in our lives can help to bring attention and awareness to our creative potential.

Sometimes creativity, especially if it's been neglected for a while, needs an invitation. Is there something you've wanted to explore? Could you sign up for a dance class, a pottery class, a golf class, or perhaps go on a day trip to a museum, a sports event, an art opening, or even to a café you haven't visited before? Sometimes simply changing our routines or our landscapes is all that's needed to awaken new neural pathways.

Even taking a different road to work or to the grocery store can bring us into contact with different sights and sounds, taking us out of our patterned mode and allowing our senses to reawaken.

What is one change you would like to make today? It could be listening to a radio station you've never listened to before, ordering something to eat that you haven't tried before, wearing something that's shifted to the back of your closet, taking your morning walk in a different direction, or exploring any other new experience that comes to mind.

Don't be surprised, however, if there is resistance. The mind is very good at becoming attached to what is familiar. Take your time. Go slowly. Or, just dive right in!

ॐ Digestion Central:
Maṇipūra Chakra

At the center of our being resides the navel—symbol of our entry into this world, this life. Through the umbilical cord came our initial nourishment, delivered to us by the divine architecture of our physiological design. In our adult life, the task of nourishment is ours; whether we offer ourselves healthy foods, healthy attitudes, and healthy experiences is up to us. Eating nourishing food and taking top-quality supplements, however, is going to have limited benefits if the body is unable to absorb, assimilate, and digest the nutrients properly.

Similarly, when we do not allow time and space to digest our emotions, toxic build-up accumulates, impeding the physiological processes. The fire of *tapas*, disciplined challenges that allow us to burn through the stagnation of our blockages, can support *maṇipūra chakra*.

The healthier our digestion is, the healthier our overall system is, and the better the chances are of us maximizing our personal potential as we interact in the world.

The warm yellow of the sun is often the color associated with this ten-petaled *chakra*, and this life-giving light, when in balance, supports well-being. When the light, or fire, is weak, however, digestion suffers. Conversely, too much of a good thing can be troublesome. Overstimulation in this area can lead to hyperacidity, indigestion, and heartburn.

When we think of all the environmental factors, from mold to bacteria to pesticides to microwaves, it's a wonder that we receive and digest as much nourishment as we do. Similarly, toxins like competitiveness, jealousy, fear, doubt, and misunderstandings that run rampant can compromise the system, triggering psychological maladies and affecting the gastrointestinal tract.

This life, with its many challenges, is often a lot to digest. One of the best things we can do, Ayurvedically speaking, is to protect our *agni*, our digestive fire. One of the ways we can do this is waiting until we are actually hungry to eat—and then not overeating. Another way to support our *agni* is to remain dedicated to our practices (yoga *āsana*, *prāṇāyāma*, meditation). Practicing daily is like putting money in the Bank of *Maṇipūra*, with continuous dividends paid regularly in the form of healthy golden energy at *maṇipūra chakra*.

ॐ The Heart of the Matter:
Anāhata Chakra

What is at the heart of the matter? At the midpoint of the seven *chakras* is the central fourth *chakra, anāhata.* Whereas the anatomical heart is responsible for pumping blood through our bodies, the heart *chakra* operates at the subtle energy level, processing our emotions. Sadness, joy, fear, anger, love, worry, anticipation, relief— all of these and more filter through the twelve petals at the heart.

Often imbued with green, the color of growth, this *chakra* governs our ability to offer compassion to others—and ourselves. By accepting ourselves with grace and forgiveness, our ability to understand and appreciate others expands. When *anāhata* is healthy, our heart center is open to embrace—embracing new people, new possibilities, and new ideas.

However, when *anāhata* is weak, hurt, losses, resentments, and grief can accumulate. Although emotional memories can stagnate in any cell of the body, the most common place is perhaps the heart *chakra.* Breathing into this *chakra,* we may feel ease, strain, heaviness, or other qualities, depending upon what is dwelling there.

We can choose to welcome love to the chambers of our heart or to bolt the doors and close the shutters. This is a choice life delivers to us on a moment-by-moment basis. Shifting the energy takes time, but as we soften into forgiveness, the twelve green petals of *anāhata chakra* begin to hum and shine. Welcoming a song into our heart can allow this *chakra* to flourish and blossom.

What is something you love? Not just like, but *love*? It could be a color, a place, a person, an art form, the Divine, a sport, or something else. Whatever it is, this is your plug-in to *anāhata.* Engaging with the source of your love plugs you into the sweetness of the nectar of the lotus of the heart. Allow yourself this love.

Sometimes in the midst of work and bills and expectations of family and friends, we skip love, bypassing what has the power to nourish our lives most. Thinking of your life as a *Namaskāra,* a salutation, to Love, what will you do today to serve and honor Love?

ॐ Bridge Between Head and Heart: *Vishuddha Chakra*

At our throat, sixteen blue petals pulsate. This is where the sixteen Sanskrit vowels reside. What word can be made without a vowel? If vowels are the life force of language, *vishuddha*, then, governs our expression. If this *chakra* is weak, we might have trouble finding words to communicate what's in our mind or heart. Due to trauma, we might have fear or sadness blocking this *chakra* and our ability to speak freely. On the other hand, if this *chakra* is overactive, we might over-share. A healthy fifth *chakra* allows us to communicate with integrity, discerning what to share when and with whom. Each time a genuine word is spoken, this *chakra* strengthens. In contrast, when we swallow our hurt instead of expressing it, we can feel a lump in the throat.

Consider for a moment—are the words in your mind in alignment with the self that you present to the world? Consider also the internal cosmos. Are there truths, residing inside, whether memories, recent experiences, or future ambitions that you have not fully embraced within yourself?

Allowing truth to flow may remove stagnation in the throat and thyroid area as well as throughout the bodily system. Expressing truth, especially about difficulties, is something that can take practice, ideally in a safe and supported environment. Try looking into the eyes of someone you trust and speaking a truth, sharing something that you have not spoken before. This can be a memory, a point of view, a habit you're struggling with, a regret, a fear, or whatever you feel led to delve into. Notice what you feel— physically, mentally, emotionally—during this experience.

If this feels too overwhelming, you might start first with journaling this truth. Finding the courage to write these words can bring clarity and focus to this subject matter residing in you at the cellular level. Figuring out how to translate an emotion, thought, or experience that's been kept inside for a period of time can be quite a feat. Take your time. Breathe. Hum. Sing. *Vishuddha*, the blue bridge between head and heart, will carry you.

ॐ Transcending Duality:
Ājñā Chakra

Ājñā chakra, located slightly above and between the eyes, is often called the third eye. In this central space that is neither right nor left, non-duality blooms. In the transformation from *either/or* to *both/and*, new perspectives and possibilities emerge. This is the center of intuition, where insight moves beyond logic, bringing forth knowledge born of heart, mind, and soul, rather than the intellect alone. Intuition, nourished by time spent in quiet meditation, self-study, and prayer, can sometimes seem elusive; however, it is something experienced by all people in varying degrees.

For instance, think of a time when you felt guided to say or do something without knowing why, only to understand later when more information about the situation became available. Intuition can come in the form of a dream, a vision, a presentiment, a sense of déjà vu, or simply a feeling. Sometimes the wisdom of the body can be a powerful resource in understanding the ways that intuition moves beyond logic. For example, recall a time when you felt uneasy even though there seemed to be no cause for alarm and later you found out that something was awry. This is the body's innate intelligence at work, picking up on signs that the logical brain might dismiss. In fact, often we do dismiss our intuition, especially when it seems to contradict what data from the "real world" is telling us.

What is the "real world"? Is it the data of science? Is it what we can see, touch, and hear? Are intangible things that cannot be measured also real? As our sixth *chakra* opens and we connect more with our intuition, our understanding and appreciation of what is "real" may shift.

This center also correlates to the pituitary and pineal glands, which are vital forces in our growth, development, and mental/emotional well-being. When we rest the forehead on the ground in *Bālāsana*, (Child's Pose), we stimulate the acupressure (*marma*) point of *Ājñā*, also called *Sthapanī*. Given that children tend to be incredibly fluent in intuition, the resonance of *Bālāsana* to *ājñā chakra* is one of grace. To walk this earth with both the faith of a child and the wisdom of experience is to integrate the best of both worlds.

ॐ Skylight to the Stars:
Sahasrāra Chakra

At the top of the skull radiates the *chakra* of 1,000 petals—*sahasrāra*. This is the sacred space where the individual merges with the cosmos in an alchemy of purification. Like a drop of water merging with the sea, we become one with the Divine.

In what way can we become part of the cosmic ocean of love surrounding us? As there is a letting go of shore, a letting go of what is familiar and what is secure, we release into the unknown, buoyed by our faith, allowing the waves of the Divine to wash over us. When we are able to rest in the arms of the Divine, supreme peace comes. The bliss of surrender is profound. It transports us from the boundaries and limitations that we often impose upon ourselves, sometimes without even realizing it.

We can sample this delicious nectar by dedicating ourselves to *japa*, (repeated chanting of a *mantra*), a prayer, or an affirmation. As the vibration cleanses and clears, the lotus flower centered above the crown of the head begins to flourish. If our *sushumṇā*, our central channel, is a tall ghee candle, the seventh *chakra* opening is the wick being lit, its sacred flame glowing, diminishing the surrounding darkness, bringing a resonance of beauty and peace.

ॐ *Chakra* Song

Seven centers of light,
you sing in us,
our central channel
alive with your presence,
you, beyond our full grasp,
like galaxies spinning in our midst.
Red, orange, yellow, green,
blue, indigo, shimmering violet,
you fill us with color, flowering
into four petals, six petals, ten petals,
twelve petals, sixteen petals,
a thousand petals, beyond—
from the root to the crown,
your wisdom resounds—
the city of jewels,
the unstruck sound,
the third eye,
the etheric anatomy
you thread through
as subtly as the breath
humming inaudibly,
synchronizing our systems,
expanding our consciousness
beyond what can be seen or measured,
you, with your seven centers of light,
a language untranslatable as the sea, the stars,
you grace us
with each petal
of your presence.

ॐ *Chakra* Meditation

Mūlādhāra, root *chakra*.
What do you root into on a regular basis?
Which parts of your life nourish and support you most?

Svādhiṣṭhāna, pelvic region.
What is the flow of your life like?
Where does your creative force express itself?

Maṇipūra, navel.
What experience in your life needs further digestion?
What in your life could benefit from the fire of transformation?

Anāhata, heart.
What colors or textures do you observe in your heart right now?
What makes your heart shine?

Vishuddha, throat.
What is the truth for you in this moment?
What have you been longing to say?

Ājñā, third eye.
What is the source of your intuition?
What can you see when you look within?

Sahasrāra, crown *chakra*.
What exists beyond yourself?
How does it feel when your consciousness expands?

ॐ *Yoga Namaskāra*

You, both sun and moon, both earth and sky,
you with your waters unending,
you of the five elements, the eight limbs,
the seven *chakras*, the 72,000 *nāḍīs*,
the infinite number of blessings unfurling
even as we stand still as a Mountain,
as we root into the floor on one leg like a Tree,
as we, Warrior-like, look directly into life's challenges,
as we surrender, resting forehead on the floor,
with the faith of a Child,
as we invert our view in a Standing Forward Fold,
as we, like a Corpse, allow the eyelids to close,
you with the ways you thread the breath
through the smallest spaces within,
the way you rinse our organs,
our neural pathways, our veins, our old habits
clean

You, without saying a word,
without claiming or disclaiming,
align us,
yoking our light and shadow,
our yes and no,
our suffering and our health,
our acceptance and resistance,
delivering us to our true nature, our center,
the song residing in the depth of our heart

EXPLORING FURTHER
Yoga's Sister Sea: Āyurveda

. . . .

A Taste of Āyurveda

When you go out to eat with a group of people, how often does every person order the same meal from the menu? Typically, due to our unique configurations, we are drawn to different tastes, both literally and metaphorically. Āyurveda, in its ancient wisdom, encourages us to examine everything from our food cravings to our digestive fire (*agni*) to the appearance of our tongue and provides methods to custom-design an individual's menu of well-being based upon what will be most nourishing, beneficial, and therapeutic, supporting the balance of mind, body, and spirit.

Āyurveda, a medical science from India that is over five thousand years old, considers health to be not just the absence of disease but the well-being of body, mind, and spirit. For instance, if your lab reports are excellent but your mind is agitated or depressed, or your relationships are not in balance, the picture of health is not complete; therefore, Āyurveda approaches each person as a unique individual and the path to well-being as similarly unique. Through in-depth questioning and careful observation of specific qualities in individual consultations, Ayurvedic health practitioners and Ayurvedic physicians explore the nature of imbalances in the body and can bring forth awareness of the relationship between diet, lifestyle, and well-being, as well as how this relationship affects the overall balance of mind, body, and spirit.

Some of the many different ways that Āyurveda supports well-being include:

- healthy eating (foods to support doshic balance of *Vāta*, *Pitta*, *Kapha*)

- healthy lifestyle (daily routine, finding balance, reducing stress)

- yoga and meditation (to support doshic balance of *Vāta*, *Pitta*, *Kapha*)

- Ayurvedic herbs (to mitigate doshic imbalance)

- topical treatments (herbal pastes, soothing warm oil treatments, and gentle acupressure)

- *pañchakarma* (five-part purification process)

Five Elements

....

According to Āyurveda, the world, from nature to the human body, is composed of five elements—ether, air, fire, water, and earth. These five elements are known as the *pañcha mahābhūta*.

ॐ Ether: Outer Space Within

Gazing up at the night sky, what do you perceive? Even beyond the moon and the stars we can travel, the imagination carrying us into the vast realms of galactic space. Space, seemingly ever-elusive, ever-widening, is right here, too, between our very hands. It is also present in subtler forms, such as the space between two thoughts or two breaths.

The presence of space within our own planet and beyond—as well as within the parameters of our physical form—is profound. Even at the microscopic levels of our beings, we have intercellular space and intracellular space. Expanding this concept further, we can become aware of the spaces we have within, such as synaptic space, the abdominopelvic cavity, the thoracic cavity, and so on, as well as pockets of external space, such as the space we have between ourselves and others.

Although space is essential, a relationship with our environment is important as well, so it's a matter of finding a balance between the two. If you've grown up in a city where you were surrounded by tall buildings with your neighbors residing just inches away, you likely have a very different sense of space than one who has grown up on a prairie or in the desert. To some, space signifies loneliness and fear, whereas to others it symbolizes expansiveness and freedom.

Do you feel like you need more space or less space in your life? Internally, externally, or both? When we feel crowded or overrun by thoughts, worries, and expectations, we can often find spaciousness by placing our attention on the breath. If there is pain in the body, it may be from constriction or stagnation. Allowing space mentally and emotionally for the pain to expand and dissolve can bring relief. On the other hand, if we feel too "spacey," we can also ground ourselves by following our breath and doing yoga poses seated or lying down, connecting us with the earth.

As we continue our practice, we may find that the space between one thought and the next begins to lengthen when we bring ourselves into meditation or *āsana*. We may also find that our reactivity to triggering situations off the mat diminishes. Having adequate space in our lives allows us to function optimally. Then again, an experienced meditator can often find sufficient spaciousness even in the midst of a bustling crowd. For now, we can start where we are, noticing the distance between our feet and hands each time we place them on the mat, as well as both the finite and infinite space that exists within, and between ourselves and every other human being.

ॐ Exploring the Space Within

The breath ebbs and flows,
the space of the heart widening,

allowing a forgiveness,
even a millimeter of space—

space in the mind expanding,
making room for a new point of view,

the space in the stomach full-to-capacity
or with plenty of room to digest—

the space between each vertebra,

the space between two thoughts,

the space, the pause, between inhale and exhale,

the space born when tense muscles
relax, the release of stagnation,

the vibration of compassion
shaping the ever-shifting space

between mind and heart

ॐ Air: The Wind Within

To rest on the ground and look up at leaves fluttering is to see the delicacy and grace of the wind in motion. From gentle sea breezes to tremendous gales, the wind is a potent force capable of rearranging our world in both subtle and dramatic ways. Sometimes the air can also become very still or stagnant, and the same is true for the air within our bodies—the breath. Sometimes we may hold our breath without realizing it, or breathe shallowly, or in irregular patterns. The emotions, with their dramatic turns, can certainly affect the rate and quality of the breath. Consider, for instance, a time when you gasped in fear or awe, or a time when your breath sped up due to excitement or anxiety.

The beauty of the breath is that it can, through specific *prāṇāyāma* practices, soothe the nervous system and emotions. The internal air of breath is so constant that we can even forget its presence, and yet this subtle thread is what stitches us to the external atmosphere in the continuous exchange of oxygen and carbon dioxide; this thread of breath also joins us with every other living being on the planet. Amidst the diversity of existence, all human beings and animals breathe. Even the plants and trees breathe.

Placing your hands on the sides of your rib cage, feel the expansion and contraction of your rib cage as your hands move out and in. Deepen your breath. Feel what occurs in the movement.

Then, place your hands on your abdomen. Follow the movement, observing its rhythm. See if you can take in a little more air as you inhale, and then extend the exhale. Notice the quality, too, of the air surrounding you and the air moving through you. Does the air smell polluted or feel stagnant, or does it feel pure and fresh?

Given that the internal air of the breath is essential to our existence, doesn't it make sense to honor the breath? *Prāṇāyāma* is one way to do this. Even simply acknowledging the breath and making an effort to tune into it once every fifteen minutes, once an hour, or while doing *āsana* can have a profound effect as the breath weaves together our mind, body, and soul.

ॐ Airing Out the Inside

The breeze moving through the leaves,
the spin of the hurricane's wind,
the breath that gave our infant lungs
a chance to begin, finding the balance
of inhale, exhale in the fluctuating rhythm of our lives,

Oh, fresh air, how you rejuvenate our spirit
clearing the stale air out of unseen crevices
in our mind and heart, a mystery breathing
in what you carry, something is in the air
we say, knowing and not knowing what it is

You, threading through every living being,
simultaneously subtle and profound,
you, a cough, a deep inhale, a gasp,
your presence, moving, circulating all around.

ॐ Fire: The Heat Within

E nvision sitting next to a fireplace on a cold, damp day. Feel the heat of the fire warming your skin. Listen to the fire crackle and pop. Watch the orange and red flames dance. Just as a fire like this can save lives by providing a means to cook food and offer warmth, it can also destroy land, a home, or an entire village. Similarly, the fire within us serves vital functions, such as maintaining body temperature and fueling our digestion. The heat within is a precious power that keeps metabolism functioning properly and allows our eyes to perceive and our minds to comprehend, yet if this element moves out of control, there can be heat-driven conditions, such as fever, hyperacidity, and inflammation.

A certain amount of literal or metaphorical heat inside is necessary, however, to motivate us to accomplish tasks and to transcend habitual patterns. On the other hand, feeling too much heat in the form of pressure or expectations can lead to aggravation, aggression, and eventually burnout. At the opposite end of the spectrum, not having enough fire element can lead to sluggishness in terms of both digestion and mental clarity.

Which situations in your life could benefit from more heat? Which situations could benefit from less heat? Watch the foods that you eat, considering their fiery—or spicy—content. Notice how often you wear red and orange or decorate with these fire-like colors. What about the heat of your words? How many times a day do you criticize, yell, or speak in a sharp or heated tone? Does your yoga *āsana* practice tend to bring excess heat and sweat? What about your eyes—do you tend to gaze intensely throughout the day, or are your eyes relaxed and receptive?

When we give our attention to the element of fire, we can begin to understand the many ways, such as appearance, health, emotions, and diet, that fire manifests in ourselves and others. From the single flame of a candle to an entire forest ablaze, fire, in its many humbling forms, transforms us and our world with its heat and power, its beauty and light.

ॐ Dance of Fire

You, with your love, your anger,
the fire dancing in your eyes,
the heat of your thoughts,
your tongue a flame,
the brilliant red, orange, gold
fiery in its simple presence,
igniting desire
to understand, to enjoy,
to create change,

the warmth in you,
your face, your words, your aura—
radiant, cooking and digesting
the delicious meal of life,
your fire, your divine fire,
your light, your dance, your heat,
your heart, your choice, your peace,
your power.

ॐ Water: Rivers Within

In this moment, rivers are coursing through us, traveling within the mind, the heart, the arms and legs, the spirit. They are humble rivers, quietly tending to their duties of carrying thoughts, feelings, and nutrients. There are rivers of plasma, rivers of capillaries; there are rivers of ideas, rivers of fear, rivers of joy, and more. Some rivers may be clogged with debris while others shine and flow without obstruction.

Bring forth the most beautiful river from your memory or imagination. Observe its rippling flow; listen to its wordless music. Consider its liquidity, its color, the way the sun or moon dances upon it. In what ways are you like this river? How might you embody more flow in your yoga practice? Which parts of your daily life would you like to see flow more easily? Meditate gazing at an image of a river, or consider listening to music that brings in the water element.

How much water element is present in you now? When there is dehydration, literally or metaphorically, the internal rivers are reduced. Lack of moisture may not be noticed until we have a dry mouth, dry skin, dry eyes, or joints that are stiff from lack of lubrication. Excess water element in the body may manifest in a variety of ways, such as edema or grief.

Consider the presence of water in your environment. When was the last time you visited a natural body of water or swam in a pool? Does a day of rain bring you joy, calm, or gloom? How much water do you drink each day? Is it hot water, lukewarm water, room-temperature water, cold water, or water with ice?

Developing a healthy relationship with water and creating a balance of water in our lives invites well-being of mind, body, and spirit to flourish, flowing like awareness through the many layers of our being.

ॐ Washed Clean

Receiving the offerings of each day, whether bitter or sweet,
with patience, with fortitude, with gratitude, we grow,
we come to know, we begin to flow.

Like water unafraid to be water, we glide, we cascade,
we surge, we recede, we cleanse and are cleansed,
we submerge, we immerse, we flood and evaporate,
we reflect, we pour and quench, we feed the roots,
we are drops, a droplet, a body of water,
a mirror of the pale clouds, the shimmering sun,
we are the rains, the snows, the sweat, the tears,
we are the bowlful of water blessed with prayers.

ॐ Earth: The Ground Within

What comes to mind when you think of the word "earth"? Do you see fertile soil, dry desert, compost, quicksand, sand dunes, grasslands, earthquakes, landslides, plate tectonics, piles of dirt, or something else? Unusual as it may sound, all of these potentialities reside within metaphorically. Just as there are minerals in the earth, minerals inside our body contribute to our bones, teeth, and nails. Our skeletal structure with its calm, grounding nature of the earth is a stabilizing force.

What else is stable within you, your life? Although nothing may be immune to change, there are certainly qualities or aspects of our life that may feel more stable than others. For instance, your finances may currently be more stable than your relationships, or vice versa. Your physical health may be more stable than your mental health, or vice versa. Your left leg may feel more stable than your right, and so on.

How stable do you feel in an earthy pose like Child? What about in other *āsanas*? Do you ever get shaking in the limbs or perhaps just in one leg or foot? Whether this is a muscle spasm or an emotional release or both, it can feel like you are having an earthquake in your body or that your body has become an earthquake. On the other hand, you may have had the sensation of sluggishness, of being depleted soil that needed to be upturned and revitalized. The soil of your heart—is it frozen? Dry? Abundantly rich? What is buried in this heart-earth? Treasures? Seeds? Losses? Fossils? What about the soil of your mind? Is it primed for receiving planting, for embracing new growth, or is it characterized by deep ruts or overgrown weeds?

Earth forms the foundation of our world; similarly, the earth element with its heavy, stable qualities is important in our own sense of well-being. When we are stable, we are better able to withstand life's storms. Our stability can be supported by having a stable daily routine, a stable job, a reliable place to stay, and steady relationships; however, we can also develop a steadiness within, even when outer supports may fall away. A regular yoga practice, when done with awareness, can help to steady the mind, stilling the waves of thought.

As you move through your day, notice the ground as you step upon it, sit upon it, drive upon it. Lie down on the ground and let it support you. Feel its steady presence. Feel your steady presence. As you travel the path of awareness, notice what happens when you bring the elements of support in your life to mind with gratitude.

ॐ Impermanent Permanence

In the earth of the mind
new ideas just about to sprout
wait for sun and rain,
dreaming in colors

In the earth of the heart,
entire fields of flowers,
fragrant and soft, bloom

Earth becoming soft mud, wet sand, quicksand,
becoming dry and cracked, quaking apart,
becoming richly fertile, ready
to give birth to new life—

we are these earths—all of them—
full of memory, possibility,
ancient mystery,
full of resilience,
never twice the same

ॐ Born of the Five Elements

You, made of the earth,
your bones sturdy, your skeleton
a well-designed architectural song,
may you walk this earth with grace.

You, made of water,
divine plasma, blood,
sweat, saliva, tears,
sacred rivers within,
may you flow through this life in peace.

You, made of fire,
flames of intelligence,
passion, irritation, anger, awareness
speaking in tongues of light and heat,
may the alchemy of transformation
keep the wick of your heart lit.

You, made of air,
beautiful devotion of movement,
duet of inhale, exhale,
choreography of respiration,
may you move and breathe
through each moment with faith.

You, made of ether,
pockets hidden beneath the skin
singing spaciously between organs and cells,
may you embrace the pauses, the gaps
in life's everflowing song.

You of the five elements—
stable and firm,
gliding and flowing,
you crackle and transform,
you breathe and move,

you pause and wait,
you, born of earth, water, fire, air, space,
in every molecule of your being,
in every thought that you think,
in every word that you say,
you are, with sacredness,
with humility,
with possibility,
a universe
of exquisite design.

Three *Doṣhas*

In Āyurveda, there are three *doṣhas*:

> *Vāta* (composed of space/air)
>
> *Pitta* (composed of fire/water)
>
> *Kapha* (composed of water/earth).

Each *doṣha* exists in all people and all beings, just in varying proportions.

ॐ *Vāta:* The Movement of Wind

V*āta* is motion. Air and space elements blend together, creating an energy that can yield creativity and imagination as well as spaciness and ungroundedness. Although we definitely need the activity of *Vāta* to move us, both literally and creatively, in this life, the overstimulation of *Vāta* can have depleting effects.

Turn inward for a moment. Where do you feel the qualities of wind and space within? Does your mind feel more like a breeze, a river, a fire, or the solid ground of earth? Each of the three *doṣhas* and five elements play essential roles in our life; the challenge is to keep them in balance.

Elevated *Vāta* can bring dry skin and stiffness, as well as constipation, while its mobile energy can lead to excessive talking and thinking, including worry and insomnia. This tendency towards anxiety and scatteredness can be tamed through establishing and maintaining a regular routine, as well as including warm, unctuous foods at mealtime. On the other hand, eating dry, crunchy, or raw foods can exacerbate *Vāta* aggravation. Frequent travel, especially in a plane, can also agitate *Vāta*.

In our modern society, the fast pace and the frequent use of electronics can greatly stimulate *Vāta* as well, causing strain to the nervous system. When we become so conditioned to some of these aspects of modern society, we often do not even realize the toll they are taking on our physical, mental, and emotional well-being. Turning off audible notifications of incoming messages for a day or part of a day can offer an opportunity to observe the absence of these frequent interruptions. Try it and see what you notice.

Choosing to reduce stress by reducing the intensity of our daily schedule can calm *Vāta*, as well as practicing meditation and calming breath practices, such as *Anuloma Viloma* (Alternate Nostril Breath) and *Bhrāmarī* (Bee's Breath).

As you move through your practice or throughout the activities of your day, observe your mind—noticing if thoughts are racing, if the mind is jumping from one topic to another, if there is worry or anxiety, or if there is a smooth creative flow. If the mind is agitated, bring to mind the image of a sturdy tree or a placid, sunlit lake. Observing the mind closely can begin to bring awareness to the presence and role of *Vāta* in our lives. Are you a sea breeze or the gusts from a tropical storm? Are you fresh air or a mysterious zephyr? Are you a cyclone or a gentle current of air?

ॐ Ode to *Vāta*

Oh, often maligned one, we would not be here
without your divine motion, your grace.
From the first moment of conception
to the last gasp of breath,
we rely upon you, in all of your light, subtle,
cold, mobile, clear, dry, rough ways.
You are the electrical impulse birthing each action.
You are inspiration and exclamation.
You are digesting and letting go.
You are the circulation keeping alive the flow.

You, Cosmic *Prāṇa*, bless us with your mobile light.
Shifting here, shifting there, you keep stagnation at bay.
You are as clear as a cloudless blue sky—not blue, but beyond,
your indigo bringing forth a flowering of new ideas.

You are, at times, a windstorm blowing the dry dirt into our eyes,
the shivering cold of a clear winter dawn,
a multitude of butterflies filling the sky, fluttering.
You are the rough bark on the tree whose dry leaves drift,
one by one, in a rhythm all of their own.

Oh *Vāta*, we blame you mercilessly
for stirring us up, for keeping us awake
in the middle of the night,
scattering our thoughts, making us worry
and cry and tremble and shake.

But without you, we would not move at all, not one step.
You save us from becoming stuck,
you keep us alive and feeling the pain and pleasure of this life.

With each breath in and out, we return to you,
humbled, offering gratitude, asking for grace,
offering you oblations of warm soup thick with root vegetables,
libations of sesame oil and ghee, a gathering of lit candles,
a drum beat, steady and slow.

ॐ *Pitta*: The Glow of Fire

The intensity of *sūrya*, the summer sun, and the heat of its rays pouring into you, soaking into the millions of microscopic mouths of your skin, is the fire of *Pitta*, one of several energies shaping our lives. The transformation of fire activates our ability to digest nutrients, information, emotions, and experiences. When our digestive fire (*agni*) is healthy, we thrive.

The potency of *Pitta*, when in balance, serves us well, allowing us to shine. When our minds are luminous, we comprehend with ease. *Pitta*, when out of balance, however, can manifest in impatience, irritation, envy, criticism, and anger. On the physiological level, it can show up in the body as inflammation, fever, and other heat-driven situations, such as acid indigestion.

Cooling foods, such as coconut, cucumber, and cilantro, calming thoughts, cooling colors, such as pastels, blues, and purples, and cooling breaths, such as *Shītalī* and *Shītkāri*, can help to soothe aggravated *Pitta*.

Bring to mind a situation, internal or external, that feels really heated. What is at the root of this fire? Can you see what started it? What feeds it and allows it to spread? Where do you feel this heat—your mind, your heart, or somewhere else? Infuse a cool blue light into this area. Breathe. Observe what you feel.

In contrast, is there something—a situation, a part of your body, or an emotion—that feels dull or cold? Touch this, metaphorically, with a flame of fire activating the possibility of transformation.

Make peace with your fire. Respect your fire. Dance with the ever-changing nature of fire, one moment at a time.

ॐ Ode to *Pitta*

Oh, fiery fire, heat of the sun
emanating from the core of the earth,
warming our solar plexus, waking the flames
of hunger, we bow to your transformative power.

You help us digest what our eyes and minds take in
You are the alchemy converting food into the divine fuel
keeping us renewed.

You, with your crackling flames, burn us,
the *tapas* cleansing the toxins of the cells
in our heart, our mind, our lymph, our bones,
our blood, our nerves, our spirit.

Resistant as we are in our ignorance, our denial,
our confusion, our ingrained habits, you do not relent.

Flame by flame, you lick us clean.

Great deliverer of heat, you send us
rashes and fevers and sunburns and boils,
anger and competitiveness and criticism,
all delivered like a pile of hot peppers
on the platter of life to remind us,
to warn us, to help us see the fire we carry

from the piercing look to the sharp tongue
to the ability to transform completely
into one who tends the fire wisely.

Oh *Pitta*, your paradoxes confound us, expanding our minds
to see the oily and liquid facets of your sour, pungent self.

Sometimes, in the intense bright heat
of a summer day at high noon,
we think we know you. We may even silently
try to escape you as we duck into shade
and dream of ice cream.

But let us not forget the work you do
behind the scenes, sharpening the mind,
keeping the pink in our cheeks,
the brightness in our eyes,
courage in our hearts,
the pure radiance of our beings shining forth.

ॐ *Kapha:* Serenity of Earth and Water

How often do you embrace life—or yourself—or your practice—with compassion, peace, forgiveness, and love? These flowing, nourishing qualities are the wellspring of *Kapha.* These calm, sweet qualities help keep the fire of *Pitta* and the mobility of *Vāta* in check, and yet, in excess, *Kapha* can slow us down and cause blockages.

If *Kapha* moves to excess, it can manifest in a variety of ways, such as high cholesterol, weight gain, and lipomas. Eating heavy foods like cheese, meat, and ice cream can increase *Kapha.* A sedentary lifestyle can also increase *Kapha,* as can sadness and grief. To reduce *Kapha* accumulation, brisk exercise is often needed. Eating spicy foods and working with a heating *prāṇāyāma* like *Bhastrikā* (Bellows Breath) can reduce *Kapha,* as well as a challenging *āsana* practice. Each individual expression of *Kapha* is different, however, and is best understood through an individual assessment.

Kapha often feels heavy and sluggish. Coming to a comfortable seated position, breathe into an area of your life that feels stagnant with the intensity of the sun at noon, bringing some heat, some fire to this denseness. If the area has been stagnant for quite some time, you may not feel much, if anything. The area does not have to be a physical area like a knee or shoulder; it might be a relationship, finances, or a sense of personal power. Bringing attention to this area increases awareness; where intention goes, energy flows.

Offering awareness to this stagnation (rather than ignoring or blocking it) can help the stagnation to loosen, little by little. Don't expect a noticeable transformation overnight; in fact, it might feel a little bit like a landslide or tsunami if all of the stagnation released at once. Be gentle. Allow tears to flow or frustration to crackle. Honor the gift that this blockage has, somewhere, buried beneath. Invite it to speak, without judgment, just as it is.

ॐ Ode to *Kapha*

Oh compassionate, peaceful one,
union of water and earth,
without you, who would we be?

Lubricating our knees, hips, ankles,
shoulders, and wrists,
you allow us to glide smoothly
from moment to moment.

Moving like a sure-footed prayer,
you create cerebrospinal fluid,
blessing our neural networks.

Some may say that you are sluggish,
lazy, and lethargic,
but it is your slow, calm, steady nature
that helps us to relax.

You surround us in forgiving love,
making us forget
our piercing pittagenic properties
and vitiated Vātagenic vacillations.

Meanwhile, your memory is deep
as the ocean. Remembering each
delicious moment of life vividly,
you are grounded,
rooted in the richness of each day
without the crackling flames of drama
or the windstorms of doubt.

Instead, you are calm, cool, and collected—
sleeping deeply, singing sweetly.

Bringer of smooth skin and thick luxurious hair,
we bow to your generosity. Without you,
our tongue would stick in our mouth,

our vocal cords would not be able
to give sound to our words.

Because of you, we know sweetness,
not just cake, cookies, and chocolate,
but the smile born deep in the heart.

ॐ Twenty Qualities: Observing the Spectrum

In Āyurveda, there are twenty *guṇas*, or qualities, that describe life. They are:

hot/cold	heavy/light
smooth/rough	oily/dry
soft/hard	sharp/dull
liquid/dense	subtle/gross
mobile/stable	cloudy/clear

If we picture each pair of opposites listed above as a continuum, we can use these pairs of opposites as a lens through which to see the world, bringing a deeper understanding of ourselves, as well as the people and situations we encounter.

For instance, did a recent conversation feel more clear or cloudy? Does someone's mood, perhaps your own, feel more heavy or light? Is your day more mobile or steady? What about your mind—is it more active or still? Your skin—is it rough or smooth? What about the way you interact with others or how they interact with you—is it more soft or hard? Is your hair more oily or dry? When you wake up, does your mind feel dull or sharp? Do you tend to eat foods that are liquid like soup or dense like meat? What is your preference for a beverage—hot or cold?

Depending upon which qualities dwell in the greatest proportions in you, you may find yourself drawn to people and experiences with opposite qualities as a counterbalance; in contrast, you may also find yourself, up to a certain point, drawn towards people and experiences with similar qualities through a sense of familiarity, which, in excess, can cause aggravation.

Given that each of the twenty qualities exists in each of us, in varying proportions, it can become a daily practice to observe which qualities are most predominant in ourselves as well as in individuals and circumstances that we encounter. It can also be useful to notice our reactions to these qualities.

As you move through your practice, bring the pairs of qualities to mind. Is there a way to soften your jaw if it is clenched? Is there a way to transition into or out of a pose more smoothly? Where do you need to lighten up in a pose? Where can you sharpen—or ease—your focus?

As we begin to see each pose, each person, each experience as a composite of these qualities, we can begin to see the light of life shining through a twenty-sided prism, each facet as valuable as the next.

ॐ Light-Hearted, Heavy-Hearted

Light (*laghu*) vs. heavy (*guru*) is one of the classical pairs of opposites in the set of twenty qualities that describe life Ayurvedically. Consider the last hour or even thirty minutes. Did you feel more heavy-hearted or light-hearted? An experience may feel more grounding if it has a heavy quality, unless there is excess heaviness, in which case the experience may feel more oppressive, as if you are mired in it. If there is undue heaviness, listening to uplifting music as well as taking time to be in the sunshine may help.

Just as heaviness can have beneficial and detrimental qualities, so too can light. The quality of light can mean luminosity, such as inspiration or intelligence, or it can mean an absence of weightiness, such as being thin or having a spring in your step. Too much light, however, can be blinding, ungrounding, and can lead to emaciation.

As you practice your *āsanas*, consider where you feel a sense of heaviness in your body. Is it a stabilizing, grounding heaviness, or do you feel unduly weighed down? Sometimes returning to the breath and lightening up on it will help, as well as trying to breathe into the places that feel unusually heavy. Adding more vigorous poses or sequences of poses can also help to diminish the stagnation of heaviness.

Heaviness can also manifest from overeating, as well as metabolic disorders or other health-related situations. If you feel that you are eating nutritiously and getting enough exercise but an excess of heaviness persists, consulting with a qualified health professional can help to unravel the situation to get to the root cause. Heaviness in the mind and heart, especially if ongoing, may signal depression, which can be serious and often requires professional medical support.

Considering where you are on the continuum of light and heavy can be a way of maintaining awareness of how you feel—physically, mentally, and emotionally. You might feel physically heavy, for instance, but very light emotionally, or vice versa. What about right now—do you feel heavy as an elephant, light as a butterfly, or somewhere in between?

ॐ Movement and Stillness, a Duet

L ife is a duet of movement and stillness. Both are necessary for us to thrive. For instance, we need the deep stillness and stable quality of sleep, just as the more active processes of waking and eating are equally vital. Ancient Ayurvedic texts classify this pair of opposites as the qualities of mobility (*chala*) and stability (*sthira*).

Do you currently have a more active or sedentary lifestyle? Do you tend to travel a lot, physically moving your body through space? Mobility also can come in the form of an overactive mind and the stimulation of electronic media. When we watch TV and surf the internet, many different images are flashing in front of our eyes; this is mobility. While a certain amount of activity is necessary and useful in our lives, an overabundance of mobile quality can overstimulate our sensory perceptions, short-circuiting our systems. Similarly, while an adequate amount (and this will vary by person) of stability can be very calming and helpful for focusing, too much stability can bring a sense of stagnation.

In your regular yoga practice, is there more mobility or stability? Some styles, such as *vinyāsa* and *ashṭāṅga* are highly active, whereas others, like *haṭha* or *yin*, may feature a slower pace and longer holds. It can be useful to sample different styles to observe their effects on you as an individual. A *Kapha* individual, for instance, might benefit from a more active, invigorating style, whereas a *Vāta*-predominant person might benefit most from a slower, calmer style.

Regardless of the style of yoga you practice, the potential for activity and stability exists in every moment in every pose. Is your breath in a steady, stable rhythm or it is fast or irregular? What about your mind? Are your thoughts quite active, jumping like grasshoppers? When you are in an *āsana*, see if you can observe the aspects of yourself that are mobile and the parts that are steady. For instance, even if you are standing in Mountain Pose (*Tāḍāsana*), your heart is pumping, breath is flowing in and out, the eyes are perceiving, and continuous activity is taking place at the cellular level.

We are action and we are stillness. As we observe these two ways of being in the world, we can come to know which situations will increase our tendencies to be more active or stable, noticing qualities of activity and stillness in both the body and the mind. Every day when we awaken from the stability of sleep into the activity of movement, we have another opportunity to hone this awareness of the balance between motion and rest.

Observe: Is your mind calm like a mountain or churning like a river today?

ॐ Hot or Cold

To view fiery bubbling lava spewing from a volcano or to be in a whirling bone-chilling blizzard is to experience the intensity of Mother Nature's spectrum of hot and cold, two qualities (*guṇas*) paired as opposites in the twenty *guṇas* that shape the universe.

On the hot to cold continuum, where do you stand? Do you tend to be hot-tempered, quick to anger? Would people describe you as having a fiery personality? Do you exude a warm, welcoming nature? Or are you more cool, calm, and collected? Could you be described as aloof, detached, cold-hearted? Or are you someone who "runs hot and cold," keeping others guessing about what your reactions will be at any given moment?

The qualities of hot and cold relate also to body temperature. Often, it is only in coming together in a group, such as a yoga class, that we may be able to notice that our internal temperature setting is at odds with others' sense of hot and cold. Do you tend to shiver when others are comfortable in short sleeves? Do you tend to peel off extra layers of clothes while others are perhaps feeling cool?

Our tendencies towards hot and cold, according to Āyurveda, are determined to some extent by our birth constitution. For instance, if we come into this world with a lot of *Pitta*, we will tend towards a heated nature; in contrast, if our constitution is predominantly *Kapha* and/or *Vāta*, we will lean more towards feeling cold. Additionally, diet and lifestyle can increase the *doṣhas*, such as *Pitta* being increased by eating spicy food, experiencing a high level of stress, being surrounded by heating colors (red, yellow, orange), being in a hot climate, and even doing heating forms of yoga, such as *Sūrya Namaskāra* (Sun Salutations).

Too much heat in the system might cause a person to become very critical or angry or to have inflammatory physical conditions. Too much cold in the system, on the other hand, might cause constipation, anxiety, or sluggish digestion.

As human beings, we are never so simple as to be defined by just one characteristic. As you sit, palms up, one on top of the other in front of you, if the left hand represents cold quality and the right hand represents heat quality, what happens when the two come together? In the circuit that is you, which aspects of body, mind, and emotions, if any, tend to get overly heated or overly cool? In the flux of life, temperature internally—both literally and metaphorically—can vary daily just as the atmospheric temperature changes day to day. Within one life, or even one day, we can travel many seasons of the soul.

Four Seasons

···

In addition to considering the individual qualities of each person, Āyurveda considers the time of year, acknowledging that the heat, cold, and moisture level of our surroundings affect our bodily systems and overall well-being.

ॐ Autumn: Letting Go

Autumn is a time of letting go. Have you ever had the chance to be near deciduous trees in autumn and watch bright yellow, orange, or red leaves flutter to the ground? This shedding, leading to completely bare branches, is a gift to witness. The graceful ballet of leaves twirling in the crisp air is a sacred choreography, as is the crumbling of dry leaves beneath our feet as the crushed leaves eventually mix back into the soil.

The *arbor vitae* ("tree of life") in our cerebellum resembles the branches of a tree. If our thoughts are leaves on this internal tree, how easily do we allow ourselves to let go of these leaves? Do we hold onto certain thoughts at a time when we would be best served by letting them go? The anticipation of the stark reality of winter with its leafless trees can be daunting but can also allow the graceful silhouettes of the trees to be revealed against the backdrop of sunset and sunrise.

In our yoga practices, we can embrace autumn's wisdom throughout the year by making an intention to let go of something specific, such as a personal expectation for how a pose will look or feel, or comparison of others' poses with our own. Instead of clinging with all of our might to the branches of how things used to be or might have been or how things could be or should be, we can drop softly into what is, allowing ourselves to flow with the natural cycle of life's seasons.

ॐ Winter: Hibernation

In the cold damp of winter, we, like the bears, usually enter into some form of hibernation. This can take different forms, such as wanting to stay protected from the elements, increasing our caloric intake to provide added insulation against the cold, or sleeping more.

Just as we carry all five elements within us wherever we go, we also carry all four seasons. The winter in us is the part that is slow, heavy, and cold; it can bring peace, calm, and compassion, or, in excess, it can become lethargy, depression, or obesity.

If we tend towards the heated qualities of frustration, inflammation, and criticism, we can welcome the wintry qualities in us to flourish. However, if we find it difficult to get motivated and often feel "stuck," we may, instead, need to welcome the energies of summer and fire through spicy food and exertion. Ultimately, winter is a time for rest, and regardless of the season within or in the environment around us, there is an ancient sweetness and support inherent in giving our mind and body a chance to rest deeply each night, with the dedication of a bear going into hibernation.

If you are practicing during winter season today, consider how you might bring some warmth and heat into your practice, such as increasing the pace and intensity of the poses or adding rigorous Sun Salutations (*Sūrya Namaskāra*).

If you find yourself on a hot day wishing it were winter, consider doing a slower, gentler, more cooling practice, perhaps adding Moon Salutations (*Chandra Namaskāra*) or *Shītalī prāṇāyāma*.

Whatever the temperature or season is—internally or externally—remember that it is temporary, visiting us at this time, making its presence known, before moving on.

ॐ Spring: Rebirth

In springtime, what has been sleeping begins to awaken. New growth appears, and while we may rejoice in the bright colors and tender new petals and leaves, this transformation is not without effort. As seeds split open, seedlings must tunnel up, pushing through soil that is sometimes hard and dry. The labor pains preceding the delivery of spring's beauty may be silent, but they are there. Similarly, when we embark upon a new plan, such as going to yoga class on a regular basis or starting a home practice, a transformational energy is required.

As barrenness is displaced by this fertile energy of change, stagnation is stirred and ultimately broken apart, which may bring a watershed of emotions. These tears, like the rains of spring, can bring growth. Sometimes, if we are busy, we can walk right past spring without noticing and delighting in its gifts of fragrance and color blossoming. Slow down. Breathe. Enjoy.

It is sometimes a familiar pose like *Tāḍāsana* (Mountain Pose) or *Vṛkṣhāsana* (Tree Pose) that awakens us, showing us how an awareness of the body's weight on a particular area of one foot, for instance, can make the entire pose come alive. Sometimes it is a word that we will hear that will plant the seed in the mind or heart, allowing new growth to emerge.

Which pose will you approach today as if it were brand new?

Spring is saying *yes* to what is...and what can be. Spring is with us even in the depths of winter and the long hot summer days. Spring is when the lotus flower of our heart begins to bloom out of the mud of our daily lives.

ॐ Summer: Sun's Song

S ummertime is when *sūrya*, the sun, often takes our attention with its ability to bring a heat so blazing that it can change the color of our skin. Some people, usually those who are predominantly *Kapha* or *Vāta*, truly love summer and may think, "The hotter, the better!" Others, usually those with a lot of the fiery *Pitta doṣha*, can be adversely affected by the heat, especially if working in direct sunlight at high noon.

How do you feel about summer? Do you look forward to summer heat all year? Do you dread summer, or are you okay with it as long as you are in the shade or near a cool fan?

To feel the heat of summer throughout the year, the sequence of Sun Salutations (*Sūrya Namaskāra*), especially if done in increasing numbers of repetitions, is likely to raise the feeling of warmth in the body, whereas Moon Salutations (*Chandra Namaskāra*) offer a more cooling effect.

Do you gravitate towards heat or do you try to stay away from it? Heat can be associated with anger; it can also be associated with *tapas* (self-discipline) or even passion. Taking a moment of quiet stillness, consider where the heat of summer lives in your thoughts, in your feelings, and in your body, regardless of the time of year. Notice, too, how the heat may fluctuate day by day and during different times of the day.

Which is your favorite of the seasons, and how does this preference manifest in your daily life, regardless of the actual season?

What if the four seasons were to dwell within you in equal measure?

ॐ Three Rivers of the Mind

According to Āyurveda, there are three main qualities present in our minds: *sattva*, *rajas*, and *tamas*. The ratio of these qualities often determines how we think, feel, and act.

- *Sattva* is associated with the light and clear qualities of optimism, gratitude, honesty, and intuition.

- *Rajas* is associated with the mobile qualities of activity, excitement, restlessness, distraction, ambition, and transformation.

- *Tamas* is associated with the heavy, cloudy qualities of lethargy, apathy, and depression.

Which of these qualities resonate as being present for you most often? All three of the qualities are actually present in each of us; however, there may be one category that stands out for you.

Once there is awareness of these three rivers of the mind, you can begin to notice the types of foods, activities, and interactions that tend to increase or decrease a particular state of mind. For instance, which genres of music tend to create a more *sattvic* or calm and uplifted state of mind for you? Which types of activities make you feel more *rajasic* or agitated? Which kinds of foods bring about a *tamasic* or heavy sensation?

All three rivers are vital. We need *tamas* to be able to rest, *rajas* for movement, and *sattva* for the light of awareness.

A growing awareness of the rivers of the mind can serve as a guide, helping us notice the facets of their qualities, as well as how the ratio of their qualities is affecting our daily thoughts, feelings, choices, and actions, the three rivers of our mind spilling naturally into the ocean of our being.

ॐ Sailing the Seven Seas

F rom an Ayurvedic perspective, we are composed of seven *dhātus* or bodily tissues: *Rasa* (plasma), *Rakta* (blood), *Māmsa* (muscle), *Meda* (adipose tissue), *Asthi* (bone), *Majjā* (nerves), and *Shukra/Ārtava* (reproductive organs).

How often do we thank, or even think about, all seven layers of our being?

Thank you, *Rasa*, for your nourishment of our being. Your plasma, lymph, and interstitial fluids keep the internal waters of faith flowing.

Thank you, *Rakta*, for your blood and fire that energize us, allowing us to partake in this life fully with vitality and vigor.

Thank you, *Māmsa*, for giving us strength in our muscles as well as in our ability to embrace life.

Thank you, *Meda*, for protecting us with the insulation of your adipose tissue and giving us our curves, our beautiful shape.

Thank you, *Asthi*, for giving us hundreds of bones to maintain our structure in this life and teeth with which to enjoy life's flavors.

Thank you, *Majjā*, for our sensitivity, our ability to perceive this world, the precise intricacy of the networks of our nerves.

And thank you, *Shukra* and *Ārtava*, for giving us the capacity to reproduce, the miracle to bring new life into this world.

May our seven seas shine brilliantly as we honor them with each choice we make—for food, for exercise, for work, for play, for rest!

ॐ Eight Ways of Seeing

I n Āyurveda, *aṣhṭavidhā parīkshā* refers to an eight-limbed method of clinical assessment, including examination of the pulse, tongue, eyes, speech, physical form, urine, and feces, as well as examination through touch/palpation. Each of the eight limbs takes years of practice to understand fully; for instance, each line and texture and coloration of the tongue can be assessed to better understand a person's well-being.

How often do we look and truly see? Think for a moment about how you would describe your tongue, for instance. Then, when you are near a mirror, take a look and see how accurate your description was. Look at your tongue again the next day and compare. As you begin to pay more attention to your tongue, see what else you notice as you observe your skin, your nails, your hair, your eyes.

How often do you look beyond what your two eyes observe? How often do you feel beyond what your two hands perceive? As we open our hearts and minds, we deepen our awareness.

In Āyurveda, multiple levels of the pulse at the wrist are felt and interpreted. Similarly, by pausing before you start your work, your yoga practice, before you eat a meal, or begin some other task, it's possible to take your pulse in the sense of checking in through self-observation to see what your energy level is like, as well as your mood and attention span.

What is the pulse of this moment for you right now? If you were to consider this moment from eight different points of view, what would you see and feel? What if you were to examine an *āsana* from eight different perspectives? Try it and see.

Five Senses

....

In Āyurveda, there are five *tanmātrās*, which are sound, touch, form, taste, and scent; these are the objects of the five pathways of perception. Often, we rely on the sensory perceptions of sight and sound. However, when we can access all five pathways of sensory perception, we become more present and aware. Of course there can be unpleasant experiences that are perceived through the senses, but they, too, carry messages and lessons for us as well. As many of us are spending more and more time in front of screens, to be in touch with the textures, scents, tastes, sights, and sounds of our environment can nourish us and help keep us rooted in the here and now.

ॐ Sound: Listening with the Heart

Every day our ears are bathed in sound. From the gentle sounds of bird song to the more jarring sounds of traffic, our world is abundant with the vibration of sound.

What is the most beautiful sound you have ever heard? Was it a particular musical instrument or singer, the voice of a loved one, or something else? When we can welcome a variety of sounds into our lives, much like eating foods of a variety of colors and flavors, we nourish the palate and palette of our lives. When we can begin to recognize the potency of even the subtlest of sounds, we can observe the variations in the tone of our own voice when we are speaking to people in different contexts, noting which tone seems to be best aligned with what we are trying to communicate. As the tongue moves to different points in the mouth to create different sounds, these intuitive *āsanas* of the tongue shape our world with the sounds, intonations, and words they create.

We can also observe the sound of the voices of others. In a yoga class, the voice of the teacher will be present, for example, sometimes intermittently, sometimes more frequently. What is the volume of the voice? Is it calm and soothing? Is it precise? Inspiring? Are the instructions easy to understand? Listening from a place of observation, respect, and compassion deepens our practice.

There is an intrinsic correlation between sound and silence as we learn to dwell in the richness of a pause. When you practice, how much silence is present? If there is music playing in the background, what style and volume is it? Does it distract you or take you deeper into the practice?

As our ability to concentrate and stay focused improves, we can begin to tune out sounds and noises as we tune in more deeply to our practice. Tuning into our breath helps to support this focus, which can be used on or off the mat. And while we may not always hear the sounds that are taking place inside our own bodies within the processes of respiration and digestion, they are part of the sound frequencies we carry even in silence. Similarly, every time we speak or hum or sing or whisper or laugh or yell or cough or listen to the sound of another, we take part in the majestic symphony of life.

ॐ Touch: Feeling the Presence

In a world where global connection is possible all hours of day and night, what is the presence of the genuine connection of touch? How many hugs, for example, do you give or receive each day? By spending a great deal of time in virtual realms, we can become metaphorically out of touch with ourselves and each other, such as relying almost completely on texts in place of face-to-face communication or even conversations by phone. Of course, the style of communication that works best will vary from person to person and from time to time.

Whether we are typing on a phone or a keyboard, petting a cat or dog, scratching an itch, running our hands through our hair, kneading dough, swimming, or something else, the ten antennae of our fingers are constantly receiving information. It is not uncommon to take this capability for granted, given the tendency to rely upon the data of sight and sound. However, there is a wealth of perception in our fingertips and all over our body blessed with the sensitivity of our skin that can perceive miniscule variations in temperature and texture.

There are endless opportunities to bring our attention to what we touch and what touches us. As you walk into yoga class, notice how the door feels as you open it, how the floor feels as you walk across it, and how the temperature of the air feels on your skin. Notice how the sole of your foot feels as it presses into your standing leg in Tree Pose, how your spine feels as it arches up from the floor and rolls back down in Bridge Pose, how your palms feel as they press into your mat in Downward Dog. Pay attention also to when something, perhaps a word, a look, or a smile touches your heart. Through such awareness, we can come to better understand how this world brushes against us, painting the canvas of our life.

In a seated position, take your hands to the top of your head and allow them to move slowly along your skull, over your ears, your face, neck, shoulders, torso, hips, thighs, knees, calves, all the way down to your feet. Massage your feet with your hands. Feel the floor beneath you. Feel the breath moving in you. With the breath within you, this life you've been given, how will you touch the world? How much will you allow yourself to receive, to be touched by its many gifts?

ॐ Form: Observing the Beauty of Life

When you look at something, what is the music of your eyes as they travel over the object or image you are observing? Do you look with interest, appreciation, skepticism, scrutiny, wonder, criticism, or some other point of view? Does your perspective tend to change depending upon the object or person you are viewing, or does your approach tend to be rather consistent?

What about how you view yourself? Do you observe your thoughts, words, feelings, and actions with compassion or criticism, or something in between? When you see yourself in the mirror, do you like what you see? Are you able to appreciate the unique nature of your appearance? Our eyes, with their carefully choreographed rod and cone cells allowing us to take in visual information, guide us through our days and also our nights when the images our eyes have received during the day mix with our inner vision of imagination in the realm of dreams. Even in waking life, we have the ability to tap into our insight, our capacity to filter the data of the world through our heart center, evoking a deeper understanding, or wisdom.

As images constantly pass across the twin globes of our eyes, the eyes can become saturated with the colors and lights, not to mention the subject matter of the images. What are you feeding the mouths of your eyes? Is there a steady diet of looking at computer screens, phone screens, and TV screens? Is there an abundance of violent or disturbing images? How often do your eyes rest upon something peaceful or beautiful?

When you are practicing yoga, what is the nature of your eyes? Are they usually open or closed? If they are open, what is their focal point? Are they looking intently or gazing in relaxation? Are they looking up, down, or straight ahead? Can they look outward and inward at the same time?

One way to check the health of the eyes is to have an eye exam by an ophthalmologist. A highly trained Ayurvedic physician can also recognize many health conditions through a careful and systematic examination of the eyes (*netra parīkshā*). Another way is through self-study (*svādhyāya*) through which we can begin to notice when our vision is influenced by projections that create illusion (*māyā*). This is the profound wisdom of the eyes.

Allow your eyes to rest, to close. Breathe. What do you see? Is there any limit to what can be seen? Open the eyes. Keeping the position of the head steady, look up, pause; look down, pause; look to the right, pause; look to the left, pause; and return to center. Then, close the eyes and look within, reading the words written upon your heart.

ॐ Taste: Sampling Life's Feast

I magine a world where all food tasted the same in terms of both flavor and texture. Although many would cringe at this, our lives sometimes follow this path voluntarily to a certain extent by repetition of the same meals, activities, songs, websites, TV shows, and so on. Varying the flavors we experience can enhance the palate and palette of our lives. It doesn't take a lot of time to add one new food item each week, or to change the radio station or TV channel once in a while, but it does require the intention to invite new tastes into our lives.

According to Āyurveda, including the six tastes (sweet, sour, salty, bitter, pungent, and astringent) in our diet is important, and given the correlation of specific parts of the tongue to specific tastes and specific organs of the body, we can understand the role that diversity of flavors, as well as nutrition in general, plays in our well-being.

Which spices do you usually use in your cooking or enjoy in the foods you eat? What if you were to select a new spice, perhaps one each month, to try?

Just as it is easy to become reliant upon a steady diet of a certain type of food flavored in a certain way, it can be easy to slip into a yoga practice that lacks diversity, and while continuity and consistency have their value, if we practice the same poses and sequences over and over for years, we may be missing opportunities to strengthen, stretch, and tone certain areas. Including a different pose in our practice each day or week can add variety, nourishing mind, body, and soul.

As you sample the new pose added to the menu of your practice, savor it, noting every facet of its distinctive flavor. Alternately, you might add something besides a new pose to your yoga menu, such as a brief meditation, chanting, watching a yoga documentary, researching an *āsana*, or creating an art project based upon a certain part of your practice. Whatever you choose, enjoy it!

Life is bland only if we believe it to be, and just as adding salt, pepper, cumin, coriander, ginger, cardamom, or another spice can transform a mountain of rice in an instant, so too can our attitudes and mindset shift quickly with sufficient inspiration.

ॐ Scent: Breathing in the Aromas of Life

What are your four favorite things to smell? Even if these scents are far away right now, see if you can summon the experience of these particular aromas, one by one, through the combined forces of your memory and imagination. Aromatherapy is a pathway to healing, honoring the profound ways that specific scents speak to our soul.

Whether we are doing *prāṇāyāma*, using aromatherapy, or simply breathing, our loyal noses, which we can tend to forget about unless we're sneezing or congested, serve us in ways that are truly profound.

Most of the time in yoga we think of the nose as the entry and exit point for the breath as we inhale and exhale with the mouth closed. However, the twin portals of the nose, serving as the headquarters for receiving olfactory information, also deliver to us the aromas of fresh roses, sandalwood incense, chocolate cake baking, and other delights.

Additionally, our noses can signal a warning, such as the smoke from something burning or the spoiling of milk. Our noses, small as they are, carry the tremendous power to bring forth a memory as a specific scent transports us back through time and space. As we pay more attention to what we smell, we can perceive more subtle scents. It can be useful to reflect upon scents that you favor as well as those, if any, that you dislike or even abhor. For instance, what do you smell right now? If you don't smell anything at all, smell the skin on your hand. Smell your yoga mat. Smell the pages of this book. Smell the air. Bring to your awareness as well what you do not smell.

Today, pay close attention to the messages received through your nose. In the collage of scents that you collect, observe which ones bring you the most joy and peace. Inhale the earthy scent of the stability and calm that your yoga practice can bring. Inhale the invigoration of the fresh scent of new rain. Inhale breath by breath the sweetness of all that life has to offer.

ॐ The Rhythm of Our Days

I n a world that now has seemingly few boundaries of time or space with Wi-Fi connecting us through the world wide web to nearly all locations around the globe 24/7, the options of what to do each day and night are endless—even from the confines of our home. This means that our attention can easily become scattered, dissipating our energy. When this happens, when we respond to one too many emails or texts, when we flit from one thing to another, our *Vāta* (air/space) can get aggravated, leading to elevated *chala* (mobile quality) in our minds and bodies, which can manifest in a variety of ways, including insomnia and anxiety.

An antidote to the stress of our fast-paced society is to create a sense of routine, or *dinacharyā*, in our lives. Establishing a morning routine, such as starting the day with washing the face, drinking a cup of warm water, taking time to meditate, or setting an intention for the day—can bring a sense of rhythm and stability, which can keep *Vāta* in balance, helping us to remain calm and grounded.

While the idea of a routine can feel constraining to some, adding a bit of structure can actually be freeing. Try doing three things each day at a scheduled time consistently for one week. For example, your three things might be a morning walk, meditating for five minutes before lunch, and taking fifteen minutes to read or listen to your favorite music in the evening. Once you can do your three things consistently on a daily basis for a week, think of a fourth to add, then a fifth. You might also try scheduling your yoga practice into your week if your practice is rather sporadic. Notice how your internal rhythms respond to the elements of routine. Surprisingly, having a schedule, as long as it is not overpacked, can ease the mind. Let your *dinacharyā* bring you delight!

ॐ Balance and Imbalance

From the weather to local, national, and global events to the movement of our own thoughts and emotions, life is in continual flux. However, staying centered in a regular routine of a healthy diet, healthy exercise, and a healthy sleep cycle can help us to stay balanced even amidst the constantly changing variables.

It is said in Āyurveda that each person is born with a particular constitution and that this specific ratio of the *doṣhas* (*Vāta*, *Pitta*, and *Kapha*) can be felt through the radial pulse. This *original* constitution of each individual is called *prakṛiti*. It can be compared with the *current* ratio of the *doṣhas*, which is known as *vikṛiti*, to assess imbalances.

In our lives, which tend to have some form of stress, whether financial, relationship-related, job-related, health-related or other, there is usually some elevation of at least one of the *doṣhas*. Ayurvedic Health Practitioners and Ayurvedic physicians can assess both the original ratio and current ratio and offer a treatment plan (*chikitsā*) of dietary and lifestyle recommendations and, when needed, recommend herbs and topical treatments (*netra basti, marma*, etc.) to help mitigate the imbalances. Doshic quizzes and self-assessments are also available on many Ayurvedic websites and can provide a useful starting point in understanding your doshic tendencies.

As we practice yoga, depending on the style of our practice, we may feel, due to our doshic ratios, a sense of balance or imbalance, which may show up physically, emotionally, mentally, or all three. If *Pitta* is high, we may be too much in our minds in a yoga pose, for instance, or if *Vāta* is elevated, we may need to pay more attention to what we are doing or feeling in a pose, or to our practice as a whole. If *Kapha* is high, we may need a more vigorous practice. Considering our yogic practice in respect to our doshic ratios can help support our well-being through an awareness of balance.

Finding balance in how we spend our time, our money, and our energy as we journey through this life, as well as how we literally maintain equanimity in balancing poses like *Vṛkṣhāsana* (Tree Pose) or *Naṭarājāsana* (Dancer Pose) or in unexpected challenging life circumstances, is a lifelong practice of learning.

Stand on one leg and observe. Then stand on the other leg. Observe. Is it easier or harder to balance on this leg? Just as gymnasts learn to do back flips on a four-inch beam, so too can we improve our balance with daily practice and awareness.

ॐ Harmony and Dissonance

How often do we listen, really listen, to the patterns and rhythms of the divine symphony of this life? How often do we pay attention to the music we carry within? Think about the timing and coordination that is required for all of our physiological processes to function properly amidst the crescendos and decrescendos and the accelerations and slowings of our day-to-day thoughts, feelings, and actions. Truly, the intricacy and excellence of our internal orchestra is a masterpiece.

An orchestra could theoretically play on and on for hours or even days in a marathon of music without pausing to re-tune their instruments or rest. Similarly, we can push our own symphonic systems to extremes, and often we do, yet the quality of our harmony usually suffers in these circumstances as dissonance between body and mind begins to sound. This dissonance may be subtle at first, such as a headache, difficulty sleeping, a digestive issue, lethargy, or difficulty concentrating.

Pause for a moment. Close your eyes and check in. What has your body been expressing lately? Does your system feel like it is in tune?

From an Ayurvedic standpoint, there is a period of time in which the body's innate ratio of *Vāta*, *Pitta*, and *Kapha* begins to move out of balance, and excesses of *doṣha* accumulate in the system, seeking a place to deposit. In these initial stages of the disease process (*samprāpti*), the body can usually be brought back to balance with the support of dietary and lifestyle changes. However, given that these early stages of discomfort are easier to ignore than more severe symptoms, many people override these experiences of dissonance and keep pushing ahead.

Eventually, though, the reed of a clarinet or oboe splits or cracks, the viola's or cello's strings need to be repaired or replaced, and the pads on the keys of a flute need to be re-sealed; similarly, the physical, mental, and emotional body will need tending to eventually, and the degree of the repairs needed will often relate to how many initial prodromal symptoms or warning signs have been left untreated.

Listening with a keen ear as you move through your practice and through your day, while noting areas and aspects of dissonance, can become a valuable part of self-awareness as well as an ongoing assessment of your well-being. As you move through your practice and your day, listen. Listen not just with your ears but with all of your faculties. See what your entire being has to say. Prevention is often a more manageable process than treatment, and if paying attention and taking health-supportive action might change the course of disease processes in their initial stages, why not begin now?

ॐ Unique as You Are

Take a moment to consider five features that make you uniquely you—from your appearance to how you think to how you move through this life. Then think of five people you know well and the five qualities that make them unique. If you all were to each have an unexpected day off from work, would you all opt to spend that day in the same way? If you were to each contract the same illness, would you respond in the same way? In recognition of the uniqueness of our physical, mental, and emotional qualities, Āyurveda takes into account these variables, creating an individualized plan to support the health and well-being of each person, adjusting it in response to changes within the individual and changes within the seasons.

This approach differs from an allopathic model where a specific medication is indicated for a specific condition, such as indigestion, high blood pressure, or difficulty sleeping, and is prescribed to many people. Allopathy is skilled in its ability to respond to emergency situations and to treat many conditions; however, sometimes the medications come with difficult side effects. Āyurveda, a more gradual and natural approach to health, requires patience and commitment. In addition to addressing the symptoms of a condition, Āyurveda aims to understand the root cause of the imbalance.

Āyurveda and allopathy can often work in tandem to bring together the best of both medical systems when there is a willingness and fluency on both sides of the equation. With the wealth of knowledge and skill present in both healing systems, the synergy created when these two vast bodies of medicine come together can be life-changing.

A fusion of Āyurveda and yoga can also be quite profound. For instance, an Ayurvedic approach to yoga takes into account the season as well as the imbalances present in a person's constitution. Therefore, a single style of practice or sequence of poses will have different effects upon different people, depending upon many factors within the individual, including the ratio of the *doṣhas* (*Vāta, Pitta, Kapha*). For example, many rounds of Sun Salutations might be well suited to a *Kapha* individual but too heating for *Pitta*. Similarly, a yoga instructor using a calm voice can work well for *Vāta* but may not be stimulating enough for *Kapha*. In embracing the diversity of human nature, we come to recognize our similarities and honor our differences. We come to the mat as common human beings and also as absolutely unique individuals born of possibility and grace.

ॐ Following the Flow of the Body's Wisdom

Would you feed your dog or a friend's dog chocolate, knowing that chocolate is toxic or even lethal to dogs? No. And yet how often do we partake of something that we know will ultimately not support our well-being? This could be in the form of eating junk food, or overconsumption of movies and TV shows, especially those that may be excessively violent, abusing drugs or alcohol, overworking, driving too fast or while texting, sleeping inadequately or excessively, or spending time in unhealthy relationships or environments.

Prajñāparādha is often translated as "crimes against wisdom." What would cause someone to metaphorically commit a crime against the self? The reasons can be many, some intentional and some unintentional, and perhaps what is more important than the individual reasons is the willingness to stand in truth and awareness, observing what is taking place, for without the courage to look at our choices and actions, as well as their results, we can remain mired in patterns and habits that serve as a blockade, preventing us from becoming our best self. Just as our phones and computers often require updates, we, too, often need to update and refine our operating systems within.

What, within the last 24 hours, is something that you have said, done, thought, or ingested that, in retrospect, does not seem to have supported your overall well-being? Rather than chastising yourself for this choice, simply observe it. What caused you to opt for this ultimately unhealthy choice? Was it sadness, fear, worry, anger, fatigue, or something else? And what results can you see now that unfolded from this choice both right away and later?

If we are the accumulation of our choices, who could you become and how could your life transform if you opted out of unwise choices, starting with one each day?

ॐ Achilles' Heel

As you gaze lovingly with awareness at your true self, what do you detect as your best qualities? What do you notice as your weakest spots—physically, mentally, and emotionally?

In Āyurveda, a weak space in the body or mind that can attract illness is known as a *khavaiguṇya*. This weak spot, though it may come from trauma or a bout of sickness, is often a result of inheritance; however, this weak spot will not automatically result in illness or disease. A healthy diet and lifestyle can do much to insure that this weak spot will remain in the realm of a possibility for imbalance rather than bringing about the reality of a serious illness.

Even without the use of an X-ray or psychoanalysis, we often have a sense of where our weak spots are as we observe tendencies to live life in ways that do not serve our highest good. This could show up as a propensity to overeat or overwork or many other means of escape. We can also often feel those areas of the body that do not seem as strong or as supple as others; for instance, there may be a tendency towards tightness or soreness in a muscle or joint, there may be stagnation in an organ, such as the liver, or there may be congestion, such as in the lungs.

Sometimes in *āsana* practice, you may notice that one side of the body feels weaker, stiffer, or less stable than the other. Sometimes it is a particular muscle that makes itself known through an ache or pain. These areas may point to a potential weak area.

Pause. Considering one or more potential weak spots within yourself, take some time to consider possible routes to prevent this potential weakness from manifesting into a more significant imbalance. What is one food you could remove from or add to your diet as a preventative measure? What is one thought you could remove from or add to your mental diet? Let your Achilles' Heel inspire you to move towards a healthier you!

ॐ Digesting Life

A delicious serving of your favorite food; the arrival of a fascinating new concept; an invitation to venture into the unknown—which of these appeals to you most? What do you hunger for? How strong is your appetite for life?

At the center of Ayurvedic assessment is *agni*, or digestive fire. If the fire is too hot, there can be inflammation such as hyperacidity. If the fire is not strong enough, there can be sluggish digestion. Often, the fire is variable, creating a combination of symptoms. There are many ways to approach these digestive ailments, such as eating meals at specific times, eating in a calm environment, reducing or eliminating snacking, and eating or avoiding specific foods to pacify doshic imbalances.

However, it is not only food that we are taking in on a daily basis. In any given hour, there may be quite an abundance of incoming emails, phone calls, text messages, breaking news reports, and social media notifications, not to mention all of the experiences and conversations taking place in real time and space. In addition to all of the incoming information and experiences in the external environment, we also have a flow of thoughts and emotions. All of this material needs time and space to properly digest, but when we are rushing from one thought to the next and from one event to another, this process gets shortchanged.

In an ideal world there would be plenty of time for all of our needs and desires, or perhaps there already is. While we may not have the luxury to schedule an hour of contemplation in the midst of our responsibilities, taking even a moment or five minutes to pause before racing ahead can bring a sense of spaciousness and calm, which can be supportive to the digestive process.

Sometimes, as it is said, "less is more." Just as reducing portion size may help with supporting physical digestion, reducing what we have on our metaphorical plate may assist with the digestion of life itself.

ॐ Revise and Renew

J ust as our electronics periodically require system updates, our mind, body, and spirit also benefit from opportunities to come into optimal alignment with the present moment.

When we take time to pause and reflect upon our life, we can identify aspects we would like to revise, considering how we might renew our consciousness through awareness to bring about a greater sense of balance and well-being.

Pañcha means "five," and, in Āyurveda, *pañchakarma* is a five-faceted process of detoxification and rejuvenation.

While you may not be in a position right now to take part in an official *pañchakarma*, which requires dedication of at least one full week (and often longer), there are ways you can honor this process of detoxification and rejuvenation wherever you are.

For instance, you might choose a week to give your full focus to the kinds of foods you are eating, aiming to improve their nutritional value. You might also take more time than usual one week to rest and reflect upon the health of your life, listing some goals for the upcoming weeks. One of the goals might be to meet with your health care professional for a check-up. You might also take time to reflect upon your relationships, assessing any elements that feel toxic as well as those that feel nourishing and supportive.

If you'd like to follow the concept of a five-layered process of detoxification and rejuvenation, you might choose five areas of focus, such as diet, sleep, daily schedule, stress reduction, and exercise.

Ultimately, the more regularly we cleanse, both internally and externally, the less chance there is for accumulation of toxicity (*āma*). What would you most like to detox from your system? Acknowledge that chosen toxic belief or behavior for what it has taught you, and then begin to make plans for how to let it go.

Even in the intention for release, the process begins.

ॐ The Medicines of the Earth

There is a profound wisdom in the language of the plant kingdom. What do you notice when you observe the shapes, textures, and colors of the leaves of plants, herbs, and trees?

At the heart of Āyurveda is wisdom about the healing properties of the plants of the earth. Herbs that have been used for thousands of years are chosen for individual protocols based upon their medicinal qualities, their tastes, their heating/cooling natures, and their post-digestive effects. The effects of the herbs on the doṣhas (*Vāta*, *Pitta*, *Kapha*) and bodily tissues are also taken into account, as well as the specific qualities and actions of the herbs. The herbs are then combined in specific proportions to create individualized formulas designed to support doshic balance, promoting overall psychophysiological well-being.

If you receive an Ayurvedic herbal protocol, consider taking some time to observe its nuances, journaling about the appearance, texture, scent, flavors, and subtle sounds of the herbs, integrating their unique qualities into your awareness.

Herbs can also be used topically, such as in Ayurvedic herbal pastes and oils. Imagine, for instance, receiving the calm, soothing treatment of *shirodhāra* (a steady stream of warm oil to the forehead), *kaṭī basti* (warm oil placed within a ring of dough at the low back), or *abhyaṅga* (oil massage). These are just a few of the many ancient remedies that continue to bring healing in the stress of modern times.

As more people turn to the medicines of the earth, there are increasingly more organizations and herbal companies devoted to sustainability. As we honor and protect our environment, we protect the ancient medicines that grow from the earth and our ability to receive their gifts.

The next time you are outdoors, pause and look, really look, at all of the vegetation present, feeling the ancient lineage of these silent beings. Then, gazing at one leaf or a plant or tree for as long as you like, read in its shape the message of its divine presence, its beautiful symmetrical design.

ॐ The Palette of Our Lives

The color wheel, replete with the visual delights of reds and yellows, greens and blues, orange, pink, purple, and seemingly infinite combinations of these hues, is a symbol of the beauty that exists for us, even in the most mundane settings. Simply meditating on just one shade of one color can be profound. When we are reminded that blue is not just blue, but royal blue, pastel blue, navy blue, turquoise, cerulean, and other shades, we can appreciate the layers that exist in this life.

Begin to notice the colors that surround you. What colors do you typically eat? What colors do you tend to wear? What are the predominant colors in the spaces where you spend the most time? Sometimes the effect of colors can be difficult to discern, especially when there are long-standing patterns. If you are interested in exploring this realm, you might change the colors of the décor in a specific room or in your clothes for a period of time to see what changes, if any, you observe. You might start simply by changing the color of a blanket or bedspread or adding variety to the colors of the foods you eat.

If you don't feel inclined to change the colors of your surroundings, you might begin to observe the colors of your thoughts and emotions. Which ones tend to burn or crackle like red, yellow, or orange tongues of flame? Which ones are peaceful pastels? Which are bold shades of blue, gold, purple, or red? Which are fluorescent or muddy mixtures? By assessing the internal colorscape, we can hone our awareness of what is taking place beneath our skin, which, in time, may lead to us being more comfortable in our own skin.

In the meantime, paying attention to the color of the sky, the color of the mug in your hand, the feathers on the bird that flies past, the shade of the color of the eyes, hair, and skin of the one standing before you, the color of your yoga mat, the colors of the words you almost said but didn't, delivers a continual flow of awareness.

ॐ A Constellation of Healing

When was the last time a comment or situation "got under your skin"? Do you tend to be "thin-skinned" emotionally, or do stressful experiences tend to roll off your back? Our skin, in addition to its protective properties, receives the benefits of healing oils, salves, ointments, and pastes through its microscopic pores. Our skin is also a constellation of *marma* points, which, with gentle acupressure, can bring relaxation, supporting physical, mental, and emotional well-being.

Just as in Chinese medicine, where there are specific acupuncture points that are related to specific organs and bodily systems, the Ayurvedic *marma* points are part of a highly complex physiological system; in fact, many of the acupressure and *marma* points are the same. In *marma* therapy, however, needles are not used; instead, gentle pressure of the fingertips is used on the head, face, shoulders, neck, back, torso, arms, hands, legs, and feet on a fully clothed individual. This is a deeply relaxing experience.

There is also a correlation between *marma* and yoga. Giving pressure to different parts of the body in different *āsanas* activates *marma* points, and, as a result, certain poses may feel especially relaxing and calming. As you move through your practice, notice the points where your skin presses into the earth or into another part of your body. Just as every point of light in the sky is often part of a family of points of light, the *marma* points on our body are unique and part of a constellation as carefully and lovingly designed as the rest of our psychophysiology.

If you'd like to explore *marma* further, please see *Marma Points of Ayurveda* (Lad and Durve 2008, listed in the Bibliography).

ॐ Radiating Peace, Love, and Light

If you were to draw a wide sphere around you, what—both seen and unseen—would be contained within? What is the relationship we share with the many manifestations of the five elements?

Agni hotra is a traditional Vedic ritual of making an offering of rice to a small fire fueled by ghee and cow dung in a copper vessel at sunrise and sunset. It is said that this offering creates a healing vibration for miles, benefitting the environment from plants to animals to human beings. While some people will embrace this possibility, others may not. However, the idea of being aware of the energy that emanates into the radius around us is a potent one.

Think about a time when you observed someone in a post office, grocery store, or airport and gained a sense of their attitude simply by watching their facial expression and body language. We are constantly entering energy fields of people, machinery, electronics, and more. At the same time, we are bringing our own energy field of thoughts, feelings, memories, and expectations into the mix.

Which qualities are currently in the radius around you? See if you can observe them without judging them. Just notice them, considering what has brought them into your field of awareness. Breathe. Which qualities are you exuding into the atmosphere through your thoughts and emotions?

As you move through your practice, what do you notice radiating from the core of the essence of each *āsana*? What do you notice radiating from your cells, your muscles, your bones, your nerves, your mind, your heart?

Let the gentle flame of awareness be present at the center of your heart, your mind, bringing to each moment a sacred offering of light.

ॐ Inviting Sweetness

L ike the flower petals, fruits, and special foods that might be offered at a *pūjā* (sacred ceremony), the sweet flavors and fragrances of peace, compassion, and love that we share with others are a way of bowing to the divine creation of this life, offering gratitude for our chance to participate in this ceremony of life that begins with our first inhale and ends with our last exhale. The sweet blessing of a gift of devotion is something we can invite into our daily lives. Every morning, we have the opportunity to choose acts of kindness and the words of love we'd like to offer as we move through the day.

Too often we may mistake day-to-day events as ordinary or inconsequential when really there is, at the heart of every moment, a sacredness that becomes available to us when we discard the armor around our soul and allow ourselves the sweetness that resides within the vulnerability of authenticity, letting go.

Even thinking sweet, loving thoughts is a way to raise the vibration of our internal circuitry and the energy field around us. It can be difficult to do this, though, when faced with very bitter, sour, or pungent people or experiences, and certainly each flavor and taste has its place and value. When we allow ourselves to experience pungency or bitterness or sourness authentically rather than covering these natural aspects of life with a false sweetness, we have a chance to taste the full texture of life. There is a time and a place for everything; by bringing attention to the role of sweetness in our lives, as well as the ratio of sweetness to the other flavors, we can open into a more satisfying, nourishing, and genuine balance and experience of life.

In the sweetness of this silence, pause for a moment, tasting the nectar, slowly, fully, one slow, gentle breath at a time.

ॐ Coming Back to Life

I n this moment, what is your current stress level? Do you feel tranquil as a windless lake, or do you feel like a storm at sea? Over time, stress can wear away at us in both subtle and obvious ways, eroding our sense of well-being.

In Āyurveda, a rejuvenative therapy (*rasāyana*) encompasses specific herbs as well as nourishing protocols and supportive treatments. In daily life, we also have the opportunity to rejuvenate as each of our thoughts and actions can lead us towards straining our systems or allowing our mind, body, and spirit to rest. Whether it is a short walk in the fresh air, a warm bath by candlelight, taking fifteen minutes to close your eyes and listen to your favorite music, or eating a delicious, nutritious meal, there are many ways that you can nourish yourself, supporting your natural glow (*ojas*) of well-being, which supports your vitality and your immunity.

We can also use this awareness of revivification to help us make choices throughout the day, such as asking, "Is taking this action right now going to deplete or rejuvenate me?"

And while we can't always opt out of potentially depleting experiences, beginning to notice their effects can help us to navigate them more adroitly, potentially limiting them and reducing their impact. The more we that we nourish ourselves, the more we have to give to others.

If we are coping with significant levels of stress, we might choose to offer ourselves the gift of a restorative yoga practice now and then to experience the pleasure and nourishment of resting deeply in supported postures as we explore the deep layers of relaxation that yoga can bring. We can also choose to pause in between *āsanas*, receiving the gifts of each pose fully, nourishing ourselves at the cellular level.

Pause for a moment and consider: What can you do today to rejuvenate the harmony of your body, mind, and soul?

ॐ Āyurveda *Namaskāra*

We come with our maladies, our sufferings,
our imbalances, our confusions, our imperfections,
our vulnerabilities, our tongues tied or voices clamoring,
our requests and needs written on our tongues,
in our eyes, on our hands, in our pulse,
and you, wise and compassionate one, listen.

You watch, observing every nuance.
Āyurveda, all-encompassing one,
traveling thousands of years to reach us,
you teach us with your science and your art,
bringing together every subtle layer
of our being with every facet of life's prism,
the complex permutations coming into focus
in your methodical approach,
the elements, qualities, and bodily tissues
all considered, and more,
your ancient texts thick with remedies,
individualized as a URL or IP address, no two the same,
each person, each situation
as sacred and singular
as this moment.

THE OCEAN'S DEPTHS
Guided Meditations

....

A guided meditation is a chance to relax deeply through the light of awareness.

ॐ Riding the Wave

R elax in a comfortable position, ideally on your back.
Relax your eyes.
Begin following the wave of your breath.
Feel your chest rise and fall in a gentle rhythm.

Notice where you can feel the breath.

Can you feel it as it travels your nose, throat, lungs—the upper lobes, middle lobes, and lower lobes of the lungs? What about in your toes, your thighs, the palms of your hands?

The skin—the fabric covering our entire body—is covered with millions of microscopic pores. Breathe in and out through these tiny mouths, visualizing the gentle exchange of air. Continue with this for several minutes.

Then, gently shift the attention to the navel. At this sacred point where you were once joined to your mother, breathe, allowing the area to soften, visualizing air moving in and out of this central point.

As you ride the current of the breath, picture yourself floating on your back on the ocean on a warm summer day. Feel the softness of the waves as they move along your spine.

Allow your forehead and jaw to soften.

Let the bones liquefy so that you become part of the ocean, rising and falling with the breath, feeling the warmth and brilliance of the sun dazzling all around you, and into the depths of you, immeasurably vast.

Breathe. Continue in this flow for several minutes.

Then, gradually begin releasing this oceanic flow as you return slowly to the familiar shore. Allow your breath to return to its regular rhythm, feeling the sturdy architecture of the skeletal structure supporting you once again.

Pause, thanking your organs, muscles, nerves, veins, and bones for allowing this journey.

Then, as you bring some gentle motion into your fingers and toes, gradually open your eyes, returning to the present time and space. When you feel ready, turn to your side and pause before slowly moving to a seated position.

ॐ Divinity Within

Close your beautiful eyes and breathe. Do you realize how divine you are? Your divinity, created by the improbability of the union of a specific sperm and ovum generating your unique characteristics, is extraordinary. It is as real as your hands, your feet, and the breath in your lungs. Within you is a rich sea of divine cells designed ever so carefully to fulfill and maintain a variety of functions at the microscopic level.

Your being, radiant with possibility, is here for a purpose. Even if that purpose is clouded over right now by pain, fatigue, illness, despair, or some other factor, your divinity remains. From your first breath to your last breath, you are divine. This does not mean infallible or irreproachable. Mistakes and shortcomings are part of the lessons to be learned on this divine journey which is sometimes so steep that the focus goes to what we lack and how it seems we may have failed.

Breathe into any tightness where the body has contracted around a limiting belief. Be patient as this old hurt or block begins to soften and release. Tears or shaking may come. Breathe.

Once things have settled down, scan your body for divinity. Where do you sense your most shining divine self? Move beyond the logical mind, accepting that it might be in the left kneecap, the right wrist, the spleen, somewhere else, or many places at once. It may also manifest as an image, an emotion, a word, or a deep sense of knowing.

If you find yourself encountering resistance, accept that, too.

As you follow your breath, allow your heart to open to the divinity of those around you as you prepare to open your eyes and gradually return to the responsibilities that await you. Observe how these responsibilities, however ordinary, transform when you see them as something sacred rather than as obligations or tasks.

The divinity in me bows to the divinity in you. *Namaste.*

ॐ Five Elements

Enter into a quiet, relaxed state, lying down on your back or sitting in an upright position. Breathe deeply but gently, gradually allowing the breath to slow. If you can hear your breath, allow it to soften.

Inhale and exhale slowly. Both realms, internal and external, contain the five elements: space, air, fire, water, and earth.

As you maintain an even rhythm of your breath, take your attention to the element of space within—the space between muscles and bones, the synaptic space between the neurons activating thoughts, the intracellular space inside of cells, and the intercellular space between cells.

Breathe. Following the cool air as it enters the nostrils and travels down the trachea into the lungs, feel the presence of air and its currents of respiration allowing us to maintain a pulse and be present in this life. On the exhale, this air empties out and for a microsecond we exist in faith, trusting that another inhale will follow.

Next, take the attention to the navel, the solar plexus, the home of the fire that digests the nutrients we take into our body through food. Breathe.

Shift the energy of attention next to the water element, noticing the subtle flow inside as plasma, lymph, saliva, and cerebrospinal fluid circulate on cue from some unseen conductor of this brilliant almost silent symphony within. Our internal waters lovingly bring lubrication to our joints, carry nutrients from one part of the body to another, moisten our mouth, and deliver the cleansing liquid of tears. Breathe.

We now honor the fifth element—earth. The earth element can be found in our bones in the magnificent skeletal architecture of the mortal home of our bodies as well as in our teeth that allow us to chew a wide array of delights.

Breathe, thanking each of the five elements. Continue resting and observing the interplay of these five elements for several minutes, noting both balance and imbalance. Then, gradually begin to bring movement into your toes and fingers, stretch, and, if you are lying down, gently turn to one side before moving slowly to a seated position, preparing to re-enter the external world of space, air, fire, water, and earth.

ॐ Three-Part Song

We are a trinity of mind, body, and spirit moving through a trilogy of past, present, and future. We are a trinity of *Vāta*, *Pitta*, and *Kapha* moving through the three-part song of morning, noon, and night.

Taking three fingers—index, middle, and ring—of both hands, gently press them into your skin, massaging your forehead, your temples, above the eyes, below the eyes, your cheeks, your jaw, your throat, allowing your fingers to linger in any area as needed.

Tap your thymus with three fingers, and then move your hands to your shoulders, massaging the muscles. Bring three fingers to your heart and gently place them there, feeling the rhythm. Next, move your fingers to the vital organs of liver and spleen, touching them gently before moving the fingers to your hips, massaging these large joints that give us so much mobility.

If you are sitting up, you can continue moving your fingers to your thighs, knees, calves, ankles, and feet. If you are lying down, bring the three fingers of each hand together so that the fingertips are touching, acknowledging the right solar side of the body meeting the left lunar side.

As you release and relax your hands, let go of the limitation of could be, would be, should be. Take three slow deep breaths in and out.

Peace, Love, Faith.
Truth, Light, Balance.
Forgiveness, Mercy, Grace.
Children, Elders, Animals.
Earth, Sky, Water.
Innovation, Inspiration, Inquiry.
Patience, *Prāṇa*, Prayer.
Creativity, Compassion, Courage.

Out of the millions of words that exist, which three will you choose to stay close to today?

ॐ Resonance

Resting on your back, angle your legs apart so that your feet are about as wide as your mat. Allow the arms to relax away from the sides of the body, hands resting on the ground with palms facing the sky.

Follow your breath, noticing its rhythm. With eyes closed, remaining relaxed on your back, revisit the sequence of *āsanas* you just moved through in your practice, gently bringing to mind some of the poses you recall. If there is one that calls your attention, stay with it. It may be a pose that you enjoyed that felt particularly calming, nourishing, grounding, or expansive, or it may be a pose that felt more challenging, either physically or emotionally. In your mind's eye, go through the pose again, noticing how it works and how it feels.

Slowly consider the gift of this pose, what you learned from it today, which may be different from what you learn from it another day. Pause, and if you like, make an intention for how you'd like to carry this gift, this awareness, with you out into the world.

Then, let the memory, the image of the *āsana* you were reflecting upon dissolve and drift away. Feel the spaciousness of the mind expanding.

Feel your skull, shoulders, vertebrae, hips, backs of the thighs, calves, and heels resting on the ground. Let go, trusting the floor, the earth to hold you. Breathe. Allow your bones to soften. Soften the jaw, the forehead, the eyes, the abdomen, the spine. Breathe.

Rest silently for five minutes or more.

Take a few slow deep breaths. When you're ready, gently stretch before turning on your side and moving to a seated position.

ॐ Constellations of Light

As you relax on your back, allow the eyes to close. As your muscles soften and let go, feel yourself becoming more spacious, expanding beyond the confines of your skeletal structure, beyond the encasing of the fabric of the skin, the vast oceans of space reaching beyond what the eyes can perceive.

As you view the cosmos in your mind's eye, notice the constellations, the stars coming together in varying levels of brightness, forming different shapes. Breathe in the light. Breathe out the dark.

As the brightness of the stars fills your consciousness, consider the constellation that you are. Which other sources of light are part of you? Who fills you with joy, inspiration, comfort? Who or what challenges you to be your best self? Move towards these life-giving, light-giving sources as you continue to breathe slowly, gently, with eyes closed.

Consider, too, what light you have to give. What act, whether tiny or large, have you offered in the last year that has in some way dispelled a form of darkness, such as someone's despair, loneliness, ignorance, or pressing physical need, such as health, clothing, food, or shelter? Perhaps there is some pathway through which you'd like to share light in the weeks and months ahead in the form of inspiration, knowledge, joy, a home-cooked meal, or something else.

Breathe, acknowledging and accepting both the darkness and light, the midnight and noon in each of our hearts and minds, in each corner of the globe, in young and old, knowing that as the moon waxes and wanes, so too does the light within.

ॐ Three *Doṣhas*

With eyes closed, sit upright or rest on your back. Consider that within every living thing in the universe dwell three *doṣhas*, called *Vāta*, *Pitta*, and *Kapha*. *Vāta* correlates to the elements of air and space, *Pitta* with fire and water elements, and *Kapha* with water and earth.

Each of these three *doṣhas* is present in us in varying proportions, and these proportions can shift over time due to a variety of factors, including stress, diet, and lifestyle. In this time of relaxation, allow yourself to explore these three *doṣhas* within.

Vāta doṣha is associated with movement, which can bring a flow of thoughts that, when harnessed, can bring creative ideas to life. Too much *Vāta*, however, can bring distraction, hyperactivity, and anxiety. As you breathe, slowly and calmly, consider the presence of air and space in you at this moment.

Pitta doṣha, with its fire component, is often intensely curious, always seeking to learn and know something more, and yet sometimes becomes so intense that the mind becomes critical and judgmental. *Pitta* also plays a valuable role in eyesight, body temperature, appetite, and digestion, but an excess will bring too much heat to the system, which can result in hyperacidity, rash, or inflammation. To begin to assess your *Pitta*, consider how many times you've been angry, frustrated, irritated, or highly impatient in the past week. If many instances of this type of upset come to mind, *Pitta doṣha* may be running high. Breathe, letting go of judgment and criticism of self or beyond. Invite the fire element to come back into balance.

The third *doṣha*, *Kapha*, is one of love, compassion, and forgiveness. It soothes and lubricates the system with its flowing water element and heavy earth element. Of course too much of a good thing can cause a problem, and too much *Kapha* can bring sluggishness, laziness, obesity, or depression. Breathe in and out with the loving compassion of *Kapha* to consider places of heaviness that may exist within the body, the spirit, and the mind.

Continue breathing gently, accepting each of the *doshas* and their current levels, understanding that any imbalances that may be present can be brought back towards balance. Let go of any effort to try to do this right now. Drop into stillness. Release any effort to try to fix anything at the moment and just breathe. Follow your breath for several minutes or more.

Then, after resting, gradually prepare to move from the calmness of *Kapha* to the *Vāta* of movement as the perceptive eyes of *Pitta* open. Allow the body, mind, and soul to return from the doshic exploration. If you are lying down, return slowly to a seated position. With gratitude for your *Vāta*, your *Pitta* and your *Kapha*, place the palms together at the heart. *Namaste.*

ॐ The Whole in the Part, the Part in the Whole

A s you enter into relaxation, with eyes closed, be at ease, following the slow rhythm of your breath. Visualize this thread of breath running through you and every other living being, gently interconnecting each living being in your town or city and all over the world with a shared commonality. Regardless of differences in politics, finances, education, occupation, and personality, we all breathe. We are all part of the whole.

In observing others, the possibilities of what we may become are mirrored to us. Every potentiality for good or bad that exists in others exists within ourselves as well. Breathe. Acknowledging these capacities within ourselves expands our ability to be compassionate—both towards ourselves and others.

We each wake up in the morning and at some point have something to eat. We speak, we listen, we think, we worry, we trust, we love, we cry, we cough, we feel embarrassed, we turn to the right, we turn to the left, we fall asleep, we dream. Are we really more different than we are alike?

Slowly, breathe deeply, and as you breathe, pay attention to both the unique and universal aspects of your breath.

Rest for five minutes or more.

As you prepare to open your eyes and begin the gradual return to the world of work and errands and incoming messages, make an intention of how you wish to honor your divine complexity and the complex divinity of those you encounter.

Keeping your focus on your divine breath, open your eyes slowly, taking in the divinity around you, the divinity that abounds.

ॐ Blessing the Body

Lie down on your stomach or your back, whichever is more comfortable. Close your eyes. As you focus on your breath, gently scan your body, noting any areas of pain, stiffness, tightness, or discomfort. Whether we are 7, 27, 87, or somewhere in between, our body has a history. Every fall, every stumble, every jolt, injury, illness, and surgery is recorded in the databank of the body's cellular structure.

Some of these events our minds have more or less forgotten. Others are stories we re-tell repeatedly—either in our minds or aloud—or both. Do you have such a story? If so, what benefit, if any, do you receive from returning to it? Do you tend to think and speak about times when you have felt healthy, content, or happy, or do you lean towards reminiscing about times of upset, pain, or sickness? Both categories have their place, just as night counterbalances daytime, and summer is as necessary as winter.

However, when we think of our body, our health, and our well-being, is our focus more on balance or imbalance? When there is an over-focus on discomforts or problems, we can easily forget how miraculously the rest of our organs, physiological processes, and body parts are functioning.

How often are we aware and appreciative of the proper functioning of the intestines, heart, lungs, spine, mind, liver, shoulders, hips, arms, legs, fingers, and toes? Is it only when there is an ache or pain that we remember these specific parts of the intricately designed system we reside in moment by day by year?

In this moment we can give thanks for the excellence of our toes and ears, the loyalty of our cardiopulmonary system, the vigilance of our immune system, the dedication of our liver and spleen. Each time we bless the body, we support our health.

Travel slowly from head to toe down one side of the body and back up the other, pausing along the way to thank individual parts of your body—those seen and unseen—for the work they do, pausing at any points of pain or discomfort to offer gentle support.

A blessed body is one that has breath—for where there is breath, there is life and always a chance to hope.

ॐ Woven of Words

As you rest quietly with eyes closed, bring to mind the question "Who am I?" As possible answers to this question move through your mind like designs in a kaleidoscope, see which words come through. The words that we use to define ourselves have power.

Bring to mind three nouns that could describe you. For instance, do you see yourself as a parent, a sibling, a grandchild, a friend, a doctor, chef, mechanic, musician, or another type of professional (or amateur)? Perhaps you define yourself as German, Indian, Lithuanian, American, Italian, Russian, Mexican, Turkish, Japanese, African, British...

Once you have your three terms, consider which definition you would like to become more prominent in your life and which definition you'd like to rely on less. Breathe. See yourself as that updated version of you.

Next, call forth three adjectives that describe you best. Are you determined, stubborn, flexible, fickle, loyal, fun, serious, impatient, devoted, argumentative, compassionate, or something else? Once you have your three words, choose one of them to put in bold font in your mind's eye; then, choose one to shrink and fade, inviting change to occur.

Finally, summon three verbs—action words—that describe you most accurately. Do you spend a lot of time commuting, singing, jogging, swimming, complaining, creating, typing, crying, laughing, sleeping, dreaming, yelling, praying, questioning, proclaiming, or something else?

Out of these three, which defining word would you like to enhance, bringing forth the action of this verb more often, and which of these actions would you like to see diminish in your life? Breathe.

Gather all nine words together in a circle around you, acknowledging each one, and then let them go. You are all of these words and concepts—and none of them. You are who you are in this moment, which is related to who you've been in previous moments, but not bound by it.

Breathe. Feel your chest moving. Your lungs, bathed in *prāṇa*, have been renewed by your practice. As you breathe in, breathe in your best self. As you exhale, let go of anything that is not serving your highest good. Breathe in—receive. Breathe out—release.

As you prepare to move from your practice back into the world of work and traffic, pause in the spaciousness of awareness, seeing yourself and others as you are and as they are, but also as you can be, and as they can be, far beyond any expectation or label, resplendent in the luminosity of possibility.

ॐ Wordlessness

L ie down in a relaxed position. As your mind and body begin to settle, gently scan your body, starting at any place you like and working your way slowly, inch by inch, around the perimeter of your body until you return to your starting point. Scan the internal regions as well. As you move your attention to various locations on this tour of the terrain of your being, focus on what you can feel. If you can't feel anything in a certain spot, breathe into this area, and if you still feel nothing, simply move on.

Try not to name, label, or categorize anything that you may find along the way. Let go of thinking of how to describe it to someone else. If you find words bubbling up to the surface, note that, and return to the breath.

Words certainly have their potency and place, but they can also distort and interfere. For now, exist as much as you can outside of the realm of language. When thoughts form in questions, judgments, or observations, don't follow them. Let them be. Return to the breath.

Language can bring expansion; it can also bring limitation. For now, let language go. Let thought go. Feel the rise and fall of your chest. Feel the weight of your legs against the floor. Allow your abdomen, rib cage, shoulder blades, jaw, forehead, and back of the head to soften.

Enter into the silence, the spaciousness...

Then, as you deepen your breath and prepare to stretch before moving to a seated position, invite thought and language to flow freely again. Taking the nourishment of the silence with you off the mat and into your day, notice the various moments when the ocean of silence merges with sound, as well as when the oceans of sound begin to recede, returning us to the particular sweetness that only silence can bring.

ॐ Rivers of Light

As you rest on your back with arms and legs relaxed, extending away from the body, eyes closed, allow yourself to let go of any effort to hold yourself together in any way. Let your breath soften into a slower, deeper rhythm. This is the sound of your body at peace. Is your mind at peace? Begin to visualize the self that no one sees—the you that exists beneath your skin in the sacred inner chamber of your being.

In your mind's eye, see the beautiful network of veins running from head to toe in patterns as intricate as ancient lace. Then, begin to feel and see a soft glow of white light moving through your veins. Start at your toes and follow these pathways of light through your body. Notice their presence in your fingertips, along your spine, and within your heart and head.

The light of awareness is pulsing. Each cell of your body is shining like a star. Observe this cosmos of stars that is always with you silently singing celestial songs.

Breathe. And in your mind's eye, slowly trace the shape of your body with white light, the sacred light of awareness. We carry this light with us wherever we go. When you are waking up in the morning or as you are falling asleep at night, bring this light to your consciousness, feeling the stars, the rivers of light that are present within you now.

SITTING BY THE SHORE
Closing Meditations

....

A closing meditation at the end of a class or the end of a home practice can seal the practice, helping us transition back into the responsibilities of the day (or night).

ॐ Grace

T oday's practice is complete. Maybe it flew by. Maybe you thought it would never end. Maybe you feel energized; maybe you feel tired. Maybe your mind wandered all over the place; maybe it was as focused as a laser. Maybe you did a lot of your favorite poses; perhaps you did some of the poses that are most difficult for you.

The point is: you are here; you showed up. You entered the ocean of yoga and you did your best for today. Embrace that, if you can, offering gratitude to yourself for showing up, for being here, and for all the others across the country and across the world who are showing up today for their practice, too, and for the generations who practiced before us, the lineage of grace that has brought us all here.

If you are in a room with others, you may wish to silently thank them for sharing this practice; even with the challenges they are going through in their own lives, challenges they may not even speak of, they showed up, too.

If you are in solitude, you may wish to bring to mind, with gratitude, those you have practiced with in the past and those you may practice with in the future.

In this beautiful continuum of life, we can consider each person as a world and each person as an integral part of the world, this world that is not ours but one that we have the blessing to be a part of right now, as long as breath courses through our lungs, carrying us with the gentlest of wings.

ॐ Singing Bowl

S ometimes a singing bowl or a gong is played at the end of class, the warmth of its vibrations filling the room and expanding into every cell of the body. Sometimes a similar feeling can come from listening to such a recording.

Imagining that you are a giant singing bowl, feel the gentle waves of vibration in the sound of your breath. As you empty your thoughts, your doubts, your worries, your fears, space emerges. Vibrations of beauty flow through in ways that, like the language of the singing bowl, cannot be expressed fully in words. As the breath flows in and out, feel it; picture waves of light encircling you in an ever-widening sphere.

The breath, like the ocean, is abundant, expansive, the music of its waves flowing through us with endless devotion.

ॐ The Gift of Collapse

There is a precision in the symmetry of ancient civilizations and the geometry of modern society. In both yoga and Āyurveda, we focus on balance, welcoming it as a path to well-being. And yet, if there is an over-focus on balance, we can veer into perfectionism, judging ourselves without mercy. If there is a priority on keeping everything together, this constriction can keep us from being available to the vulnerability, the softness, the openness of living authentically. Sometimes it takes a complete collapse—physically, mentally, or emotionally—or all three—or at least a wobbling, a wavering, a significant undoing of our balance—to humble us, to recalibrate our systems, to re-wire our way of looking at ourselves and others.

So the next time you fall out of a pose, fall out of a relationship, fall out of alignment with the person you thought you were, see if you can view this as an invitation for transformation rather than as a failure. More valuable than the appearance of perfection is the impeccability of our willingness to encounter our full self. Through each collapse, our humility deepens, opening our heart-mind to the wisdom of both the imbalance and balance as shadow and light intertwine.

ॐ Soft Petals of Compassion

Compassion is rooted in respecting the complexity of life and in appreciating the threads of humanity that we share with every other living being. If we think of compassion as a flower, there is the possibility that it is hardy like a geranium or chrysanthemum or quite delicate and ephemeral like a rose. Is compassion blooming equally in all seasons, or does it seem to be dormant at times?

To deny ourselves a sense of togetherness with those who share the planet with us is to remove the sweet fragrance of compassion's flowering from our life. We may not be able to reduce the suffering of others, but by offering a caring awareness of their pain, even silently, we honor our shared journey as human beings on this planet at this time.

We can begin by offering ourselves compassion and grace when we fall short of our own expectations and the expectations of others, or when we are experiencing hurt. On some days it may feel easier to offer compassion to others—even those far away in other states or countries—than it does to offer compassion to ourselves, or it may feel more natural to feel compassion for our own struggles than those of people we don't even know.

Can you feel the compassion that others have for you? Inhale, and as the air enters, breathe in the compassion, the kindness, the understanding that others have for you. Notice how this feels.

Exhale, and as the air exits your body, breathe out the compassion that you have for others—expanding from those who may be in the room with you to those who may be on the other side of the world. Practice this with slow deep breaths, inhaling and exhaling.

Then, take one palm and place it on your heart. Take the other palm and place it on top of the hand on your heart, and as you breathe slowly in and out, feel the sweet nectar of compassion you have for both yourself and others, the soft petals of its peace fragrant with grace.

ॐ Charting the Tides

Yoga, just like anything else, can feel quite different one day to the next. This may be based upon the poses that we do, the way we are feeling physically or emotionally, our energy level, or a combination of these. If we take a few moments to log our practice after class by jotting down a few notes, such as which poses we did, how we felt before practice, during practice, and after practice, we can come, over time, to begin to observe nuances and patterns in our experiences of the *āsanas*.

In the present, making some notes provides a chance to pause and reflect on our practice. Later, when flipping through the notes, we can see how our current thoughts and feelings about the poses may differ from what they were six weeks or six months ago.

Just as the ocean's tides shift from day to day, shaping the shore, we, too, are shaped on a regular basis by the shifting tides of life. When we begin to be able to stay balanced in poses regardless of high tide or low tide in our thoughts and emotions, we embody both the stability of an anchor and the ability to flow like the sea.

ॐ Airplane Mode

The seatbelts are fastened, the pilot receives clearance, and the plane lifts off. Who are we when we are suspended in the air, hovering in transition from one location to the next? When we are allowed only one or two bags of limited weight, what is it that we choose to carry? What is so precious to us that we place it in a carry-on? At the airports, we see crowds of people lugging their baggage. What is it that we all carry? Even if we are not holding a suitcase, feelings and thoughts often stow away within our mind, our heart, our cellular structure.

When we are in the seat of an airplane, what remains with us? What do we reach for—a movie, a book, snacks, headphones filling our ears with music, or something else? Do we immediately begin speaking with the person beside us, or are we content to be silent? What is our reaction when loud conversations or cries of babies unfold around us? If every moment is a meditation, what are we observing when a sudden jolt of turbulence sends beverages flying into the aisle? Are we the same person when we land as we were when the plane took off?

What about in yoga class—are we the same at the end of the class as we were when class began? How much of our baggage did we let go of, even temporarily? When the plane lands, we switch out of airplane mode. Do we switch out of yoga mode when class ends? Today, invite at least one aspect of your practice to accompany you throughout the rest of the day, noticing with compassion what unfolds.

ॐ Layers

J ust as the ocean takes on different colors and temperatures at different depths, so too are the layers of our practice distinct from one another.

For instance, the first time we read an ancient text like the *Yoga Sūtras*, most of our attention will likely focus on understanding the key points. On a second or third read, we may notice symbols or metaphors, and we may begin to place one commentary or translation side by side with another to deepen our understanding. Still later, we may transliterate from the *Devanāgarī* or chant the Sanskrit aloud.

Likewise, our first understanding of the first two limbs of yoga (*yama* and *niyama*) will likely transform into a vastly different experience when we reach a deeper layer of comprehension months or years later. For instance, our first experience of *shaucha* (cleanliness) may be keeping our living space, workspace, car, and yoga mat clean, while a further layer may take us to cleaning up our thoughts, attitudes, and habits.

Similarly, adding repetitions of a *prāṇāyāma* can take us, over time, to deeper and deeper layers.

Returning to an *āsana* from today's practice, consider its layers. How did it feel? How did it feel a month ago? How would it feel to go deeper into the pose? There is no rush, just endless layers and levels to explore.

ॐ Counterpose

B ridge Pose to Knees-to-Chest Pose. Camel to Forward Bend. We twist to the right; we twist to the left. In yoga sequences, counterposes assist us in maintaining equilibrium. Similarly, we can incorporate counterposes into our lives; if we are constantly saying Yes, we might try saying No once in a while, or vice versa. If we are frequently talking, taking an hour—or even a day—in silence may be therapeutic, just as it may be beneficial to go out into the community if we are spending the majority of our time in solitude.

On the mat and off the mat, counterbalancing assists us in maintaining our well-being. We often focus on the front of the body in yoga because it's what we can see, but just as there is a backside to every pose and story that is equally important, there is almost always a benefit awaiting us when we can embrace—or at least consider—the opposite of what we can most easily feel and see.

Ayurvedically speaking, if you are very active, especially if you travel a lot, it's important to counterbalance this mobility with stability. If you are working overtime, adding rest and relaxation can bring a return of balance to body, mind, and soul.

Essentially, whatever you do often, try doing less often, and whatever you tend to avoid, such as a thought, emotion, or experience, consider opening to it, in a healthy way.

As you move out into the rest of your day or night, see where you might invite a counterpose of a thought or habit into your experience. Expanding the spectrum of our experience can help us to see more clearly, allowing movement in a direction opposite to our habitual patterns, bringing us, eventually, into deeper harmony.

Try it. Consider what you typically do right after class or practice is over. For today, try something different, in keeping with a healthy choice. See how it feels. See what you notice.

When you find yourself in a difficult moment later, see how it might feel to move in an opposite direction—away from the upset rather than further into it, perhaps by taking a few slow deep breaths or repeating a *mantra*, a prayer, or an affirmation. On the other hand, if you tend to typically run from confrontation, or space out in moments of difficulty, see how you might move gently towards the difficulty, or at least stay present, body, mind, and soul.

Somewhere between the pose and the counterpose, between the familiar and the unfamiliar, between the forward and backward, between the "will be" and "used to be," there is a union in the center, a union in the breath.

SITTING BY THE SHORE: CLOSING MEDITATIONS • *301*

ॐ Virtual Reality

As we surf the internet, moving from one website to another, some of the waves we encounter are smooth and lovely, while others, perhaps those with news of current events, may feel more like tidal waves at times. As we spend more and more time online each day, how often do we check to see if our internal system is online (or offline)?

We upload and download, giving and receiving. Sometimes the computer will give us a message asking if we trust the site we are about to download from. Yet, how often do we pause to consider the source of what we are downloading offline in daily life, regardless of whether the information is criticism, neutral, or praise? Similarly, how much care do we infuse into what we are uploading into the atmosphere, whether it is verbal or non-verbal?

If your day today were to be a streaming webcast, what would it show? If your life were to carry an attached file, what would this attachment be?

In yoga class, we come together in a synchronous environment, tilting our bodies into Triangle pose in unison. Asynchronously, people in other yoga classes and other locations at other times are also taking *Trikoṇāsana* pose. Face to face and online, our experiences are as authentic as we allow them to be.

What is your password—what word, phrase, or image opens the portal of your mind, your spirit? Memorize this, keeping it safe within your heart.

ॐ Churning

I n Sanskrit, the word for herbs that have been ground together with mortar and pestle into a powder is *chūrṇa*. This word, so similar in sound to the English word "churn," brings to mind how we are all part of a *chūrṇa*. We are a part of the global *chūrṇa*, the national *chūrṇa*, the *chūrṇa* of our community in our neighborhood, at our work place, and in our relationships. We are constantly combining and recombining with the qualities (*guṇas*), previous experiences, and expectations of ourselves and others. Over and again, we have the chance to see anew, to feel anew, as we are mixed in these individual and universal ways.

Similarly, the ocean of yoga is always churning, sometimes quietly and nearly imperceptibly, and other times quite dramatically. Debris such as driftwood, seaweed, horseshoe crab shells, and an assortment of other odds and ends can wash up to the surface when the sea is churned up by a storm. Likewise, moving and holding our muscles in specific ways in *āsana*, working with the breath in *prāṇāyāma*, or sitting in meditation can churn things up unexpectedly. And yet, just like in nature, it will settle down eventually if we allow it to. And then some more churning will occur. And then our breath and mind will settle back down again, as the natural ebb and flow of life continues.

ॐ Gathering the Fruits

At the end of a yoga practice, do you jump up? Do you grab your keys to get back on the road and on your way? Do you rush to check your phone for any messages you may have missed? What if you were to pause, just for a moment or two, or even just move slowly, mindfully, gathering the fruits of your practice as if strolling along the shore, examining seashells and colored rocks and glass that have washed in from the sea?

Perhaps the pause is acknowledging that you have completed a healthy practice, giving your best effort without straining or overtaxing your capacity. Perhaps it is realizing that you were able to go deeper into a pose. Perhaps it is noticing that your breath remained calm throughout your practice, or that there wasn't as much mind chatter, or that you were able to accept the challenges you had in class with more self-compassion.

Likewise, if there is something that you don't feel so good about in relationship to your practice, can you allow it to wash back out to sea? Whether you feel neutral, pleased, or disappointed about how your practice unfolded, chances are it will be different the next time. To embody impermanence is to be like the sea, moving with the transformations each practice, each moment brings.

ॐ Seagull's View

Flying high above the shimmering waters of the sea, gulls soar through the salt air in graceful patterns. What do they see? When seagulls spy something of importance, such as fish, they swoop in from above. In contrast, the activities of our days can consume us, and our thoughts and emotions can loom ever larger, easily creating a perspective shaped, and often skewed, by individual dramas.

Just as the seagull makes good use of its ability to zoom in, we have the ability to widen our view, taking in the whole scene rather than focusing solely on our part in it; however, this expansion of perspective can take practice.

Think of a recent situation that was upsetting. How much will this situation affect you a year from now? Ten years from now? Does the attention you're giving it now feel necessary, or possibly excessive? One way to practice with perspective is to pay attention to a specific part of the body in an *āsana* while also remaining aware of the entire body. For example, focus on the inside edges of your feet while also maintaining awareness of your ankles, hips, shoulders, spine, neck, throat, lungs, and hands.

Another way to practice with perspective is to zoom into a specific point of the body that may be weak, in discomfort, or out of alignment, while maintaining a steady breath with a sense of calm and gratitude for being within the practice. This is different from fixating or obsessing about a part of the body and losing track of the rest of what's going on. It is also different from going through the poses on autopilot, numbing out or spacing out so that the mind and body are essentially divorced. Keeping the attention on the breath will help to keep the mind and body unified. However, it doesn't hurt to become that seagull in the sky at least once a day, taking a bird's eye view, remembering that our lives, as beautifully unique and intricate as they are, are small drops in the ocean of time.

Considering the vast horizon of this life, how will you embrace the precious moments remaining in this singularly exquisite day?

ॐ Ocean Within

Within you, an ocean of peace.
Within you, an ocean of love,
understanding, compassion flowing.
Feel its waves washing over you,
through you, washing every bone, every cell,
every feeling, every thought.

An ocean of truth and beauty within.
The brilliance of sunlight dancing upon water,
and the gentle rhythm of the waves,
this beauty, this peace, alive and flowing in you.

You—an ocean of light.
You—an ocean of peace.
Your love, like the ocean, vast and deep.

Flowing through you, the loveliness of the sea.

You, the ocean. You, the waves.
You, the light on water.
You, the peacefulness washing upon every shore.

ॐ Ocean of Peace

Ocean of peace—come,
even as we are shipwrecked,
even as our lives are upended,
wash over us with your healing waters,
wise in the way of generations
witnessing every pain,
every loss, every suffering,
still greeting the morning
with praise, still meeting
the hollow of night with heart open
to song, in silence and in sound,
vibrations of love overflowing,
the prayer of peace echoing, resounding,
like a bell, a gong

ॐ Ocean of Meditation

Breathe into the spaciousness
of this moment,
dimensions unfolding,
the vastness of your Self,
this universe,
expanding with each inhalation
and exhalation,
your consciousness awakening,
radiant like sun on water,
the abundance of space,
the flow of waves,
the ocean of meditation
ever-widening, ever-deepening,
limitations of the mind receding,
releasing you into the part of you
you can't see, can't touch, can't know
except in the deepest reaches
of yourself merging
one breath at a time
with the immeasurable expansiveness
of the limitless Divine

ॐ Ocean of Compassion

Compassion, your ocean, abundant
with balm, the loving play of light
upon night-dark waves, the way
you gild unfathomable depths with warmth,
encompassing textures
of silt, glass, sand, seaweed, jellyfish,
squid, shell, driftwood, debris
with equanimity and grace,
letting it all sift through you
with divine measure,
your light equally resplendent
upon a broken shard
as upon a gelatinous jellyfish tentacle
as upon a treasure washed unexpectedly ashore,
the days turning in their own tides,
a steady rhythm of this and that
rocked by storms and disturbed currents
of ships passing through,
and yet even in the midst of drowning,
you surface, buoyant, fully aware
of the riptide's pull, a rescue boat
that does not seem like a rescue boat at all
but a resuscitating breath
arriving just as the last exhale empties out

ॐ Ocean of Devotion

Overflowing with love,
rich with ever-deepening faith,
offering each of your words
as fresh flowers fragrant as jasmine,

offering each of your thoughts
as candles illuminating
what remains to be seen,

offering each of your losses
as ever-purifying rivers
of prayers and tears
washing your heart clean,

you, cherishing what is true,
honoring what brings joy,
you, the precious one
recognizing all as sacred,
turning your face toward the light
even as your heart softly holds the night

ॐ Ocean *Namaskāra*

Moon-sung tides of the ocean, how you restore us
with one glimpse of your majestic waves,
with one breath of your salt air,
the way you rise, curve, roll, crash-flatten-foam
onto shore, the way you drench the sand
with the water, shells, and seaweed you carry in from afar,
the way you, abode of fish and whales, dolphins and crabs,
sharks and pearls, squid, eels, and sea turtles,
harbor in your immeasurable depths
the treasures and wreckage and drownings of millennia,
despite the blood and jewels you have swallowed,
you, buoyant, carry us, floating us on our backs,
face to the sun, you carry our barges, water taxis,
submarines, cruise ships, jet skis, cargo boats, water skis,
as we trace and re-trace our journeys,
leaving shore, returning to shore,
you, with your constantly changing currents and tides,
anchor us with your devotion, your steadfastness, your grace.

ॐ Waves of Love

If the ocean reflects the sky
and the ocean of yoga is within us,
within the quiet waves of our breath,
the shifting tides of our heart,
the sometimes tumultuous waves of our thoughts,
the shifting sands of impermanence,
what skies do we reflect?
What shines in us?
What do we mirror?

If the rays of the sun and the glow of the moon
translate their ancient languages of light
to the surface of the sea,
what do we, in the fluctuating waves
of our practice, interpret?
What light can we carry on our backs, in our throats,
in our eyes, in the fingertips that touch this world?
How bravely can we sing the darkness,
sacred corollary of the light?

The alchemy of grace sending the breath
swimming into the sea of consciousness uniting us all,
waves of love constantly washing through,
whether we see the waves or feel them
or even believe they're there.

ॐ Embodying the Sea

Within the ocean of the world
lives the ocean of your mind,
the ocean of your heart.

What is swimming through,
floating through these waters?

What kinds of storms crest the waves?
Will these waves one day stand
firm as a mountain range?
What do they hide in their depths?

If you were to scuba dive into your heart,
what would you find? If you were to snorkel
into your mind, what would you see?

If you were to create *Oceanāsana*
what would it be?

Sitting, lying down, kneeling, or standing,
become the sea…as a stationary pose
or moving, embodying
what you perceive the ocean to be.

ॐ Silence *Namaskāra*

Silence, what deep oceans you swim
carrying us into the bleak and the sublime,
your subtlety as profound as the echo
of a rock through which fossils still sing.

Oh, often elusive one, how humbly you bear
the sound of radio waves, washing machines,
traffic of all kinds pouring across the day and night
twenty-four hours of vibrational pull
and yet, you say nothing, the waves of noise
moving in their own tides, crashing against
shores inside and out. Release.

Then, in seconds, moments, sometimes hours,
silent, gentle like a prayer flag fluttering,
you wash clean our internal noise,
our not-knowing, distractions dissolving,
everything coming back to center,
the intrinsic song of awareness
awakening in the pause.

ॐ Living Prayer

How fully do we appreciate the daily moment-by-moment gift of life? Is our movement toned with gratitude for the ability we have to root into the earth with the soles of our feet, to reach towards the sky with arms stretched above our heads, fingertips extending, to flow from one *āsana* or daily movement to the next?

We accept the incoming breath; we surrender the exhale. We move, whether it is *āsana* or the ordinary movements of our day, in a continuous prayer of movement punctuated by stillness.

Whether we are kneeling or bowing, or arching our spine into a bridge; whether we are in silence or singing or chanting or speaking; whether we are at the grocery store or in traffic or at work, we are living our practice, in one way or another, even if it is realizing that our practice is faltering. In the midst of every moment, the sanctuary of peace is present. The prayer of our being, fed by the breath, is alive.

ॐ 108 Lines Written in the Sand

In the depths of sleep and dream,
images and thoughts wash in, recombine,
redesign our awareness as we awaken
(again), the light washing in over us,
the sun blessing us with a new day,

the waves of the ocean gilded
with sunrise's mercy, releasing us
from yesterday, all of our actions
and inactions receding into the past,

the golden streaks of orange and pink
arriving as if they've never arrived before,
brilliantly bold in their music
playing temporarily across the sky
whether we are there to see it or not,
the ephemeral gift, like life,
offered to us as the ocean
offers wave after wave,

the flow of the sea not unlike the flow
of the breath moving in and out,
shaping us even as the wind sculpts the sand,
thoughts drifting through us
like clouds of all sizes and shapes
moving through the sky, sometimes cloudy
sometimes clear, our minds awake
and alive to the possibility
of the next moment, the next breath
transforming the seascape of our soul,

each experience like a footprint
dissolving as the tides shift,

memories washing in like shells
from great distances, like stars
hidden in the daylight, the unseen guides
of night travelers who remember the old ways,

the GPS systems embedded into the skies
for eyes knowing how to read constellations
not just of time and space but the patterns
in life occurring and reoccurring
like kaleidoscopic designs of color and symmetry
originating in ancient *maṇḍalas*
and *raṅgoli* artwork appearing and disappearing
in colored sand, colored rice, flower petals
carefully, elaborately arranged

only to be swept away not unlike
the way life with its weathers
shifts our course
sometimes without warning,
our navigational skills challenged
moment by moment,
the anchoring of our understanding
unmoored by the jolts
appearing like lightning bolts,
sudden whitecaps in our thoughts,
shore receding rapidly from view,

but then the rhythm of the breath returns, steadying us,
and, returning to the breath,
we, no longer lost at sea,
have our compass, the breath guiding us,
even as sand swirls into our eyes,
sticking between our toes and our words,
the breath sustaining us as we hover

between inhale and exhale
the medicine of the pause
between sleeping and waking
between silence and voice

between call and response
between birth and death
between hello and goodbye
between morning prayers
and evening prayers

the pause, the second or minute
in between, a shelter, a refuge,
a pivot in which everything
can change, transform, revise,
renew, the eyes blinking
and opening to a new view,
a perspective obscured
just a moment ago
just as cloud cover
can disappear the entire sun
or moon for a period of time,

and who is to say
what is going on beneath the surface
of the sea of this moment,
the leagues unseen and pulsing,
the schools of thought swimming through
the hidden realms of flippers and fins,
the unheard chants, repeated sounds,
sonar vibration alive and well
beyond the grasp of the human ear,
its shape not unlike the conch shell,
the echo of the waves silently folded
into its seaborne curves, and when washed upon shore
and carried far from its source
the resonance of its essence not lost,

translating in a new tongue
the way we transliterate the silence
through meditation, everything emptying out
by drop, by wave, by sea, the gradual exodus
emptying us so that we may receive,

like the scooped-out holes children make in the sand
filled to overflowing
when the tide rushes in.

We, made of earth and water,
sky and space and fire, we race,
we slow, we erase, we try again,
we breathe, we look out at the sea,
we look in at the sea, we breathe,
we are enough, we (again) begin.

Contemplations

May the questions below invite contemplation and *svādhyāya* (self-reflection), either in silent meditation, meditative written response, or in conversation.

Go with the flow

Set 1: Yogic Path

1. What originally led you to yoga? What leads you to yoga today?

2. What are five words you associate with yoga? Why?

3. What intrigues you most about yoga in generations past?

4. What interests you the most about yoga as it is practiced today?

5. When have you felt most encouraged and supported in your yoga practice?

Set 2: Transformation

1. What has been the most challenging moment or period in your yoga journey?

2. When you think back to your life before you began practicing yoga and then consider your life today, what do you notice?

3. Which *āsana* is most challenging for you? What do you feel in this pose?

4. Which *āsana* do you enjoy the most? Why?

5. If you were to describe your experience of yoga to someone else, what would you say?

Set 3: Exploring Within

1. Which of the *yamas* (*ahiṃsā, satya, asteya, brahmacharya, aparigraha*) feels most challenging for you at this point in your life? Why?

2. Which of the *niyamas* (*shaucha, santoṣha, tapas, svādhyāya, Īshvara praṇidhāna*) feels most inspiring to you? Why?

3. Which of the afflictions or *kleshas* (*avidyā, asmitā, rāga, dveṣha, abhinivesha*) seems to be most present in your life, and in what way?

4. How often do you pay attention to your breath? What do you notice about it when you do?

5. When you hear or see the word "meditate," what comes to mind?

Set 4: Aligning Body, Mind, and Consciousness

1. What relationship do you see between your food intake (both quantity and quality) and your yoga practice?

2. How would you describe your digestion—of food? Of emotions? Of information?

3. What are the strongest sources of stress in your life right now? Which aspects of yoga seem to reduce your stress most?

4. Which of the eight limbs of yoga (*yama, niyama, āsana, prāṇāyāma, pratyāhāra, dhāraṇā, dhyāna, samādhi*) are you giving the most attention to now in your practice?

5. Which of your seven *chakras* do you feel is likely most healthy right now, and why?

Set 5: Integrating the World Around Us with the World Within

1. Where is your favorite place to practice yoga? Why?

2. What is your favorite time to practice yoga? Why?

3. How does the season or weather affect your yoga practice?

4. Which poses feel most heating to you? Which poses feel most cooling and calming to you?

5. What (besides yoga) brings you the greatest sense of calm and balance in your life?

Set 6: Deepening Your Practice

1. What word or phrase, if any, helps you to focus or go deeper in your practice? What roles do music and silence play in your practice?

2. Have you ever listened to Sanskrit being spoken, chanted, or sung, or have you ever tried writing in *Devanāgarī*? If so, what was your experience?

3. When have you experienced impermanence most profoundly, and how do you feel yoga assists you in times of sudden fluctuations in life?

4. Which of the five elements (ether, air, fire, water, earth) seems most present in you today, and in what way?

5. Do you feel that you tend to exhibit more qualities of *Vāta* (air/space), *Pitta* (fire/water), or *Kapha* (earth/water)?

Set 7: The Gift of Health

1. What is one transformation you'd like to see in your health (body, mind, and spirit), and what is one practical step you can take this week to move towards that goal?

2. If you were to give a gift certificate for yoga classes to someone, whom would it be, and why?

3. If you were to give a gift certificate for an Ayurvedic consultation or treatment to someone, whom would it be, and why?

4. If you were to give yourself one hour (or more) of time this week, what would you do with this "extra" time?

5. What is one way you could allow yourself to receive the gifts of this universe more fully today?

Afterword

Writing this book has been a surprising journey—sometimes like holding an *āsana* for an extended period of time or moving through a sequence of challenging poses, some of them quite unfamiliar. There have also been many periods of deep, peaceful stillness. Altogether, the process has been a profoundly humbling and rather intense experience of *tapas* (disciplined transformation) with plenty of *Īshvara praṇidhāna* (surrender and faith) along the way.

Yoga's ocean, though often serene, encompasses all the weathers of life. Sometimes it seems to be as elusive as the horizon and other times only steps away. Over the years, yoga's ocean has, at times, sent salt water up my nose, sent me tumbling underwater on its sometimes rough sands and rocks, its jellyfish occasionally stinging me, its riptides flummoxing me, and its undertow pulling me in, its brilliant sunlit waves carrying me, washing over me as I have swum, floating on its calm surface, and leaping into its magnificent waves.

Even after fifteen years of practice, I find that I am a beginner as if seeing the expanse of the sea for the first time. Yoga has daunted and inspired me with its depths, its mystery, its seemingly endless reaches. There have been moments when I have felt as if I might drown, and moments of ease as if I were a dolphin swimming or a gull soaring, but in most moments, there has been the sand of the ordinary between my toes.

Writing these meditations began as a daily *rasāyana* (rejuvenative therapy) to focus in a positive direction in the midst of grief. Once these daily writings began to accumulate in my notebook, I realized I was writing about the eight limbs of yoga, and it expanded from there. Yoga and

Āyurveda go hand in hand, so Āyurveda was there, too. The writing nourished me, restoring my soul, though as I moved through the process of grieving, there were some days when I was too fatigued of mind, body, and/or spirit to write and/or practice. Even as dedicated practitioners we can enter periods of great storms or bleak seemingly endless solo journeys through formidable deserts, but then there is some light, some truth that reminds us who we are, that takes us home, that returns us to our breath, and everything begins to unfold.

So whether you are right at the heart of the center of your well-being on a regular basis or whether you are at the furthest periphery, or somewhere in between, there is another day coming which may be quite similar to this day or more different than you could ever imagine. Breathe. Feel the tides of the ocean ebb and flow. Look up at the sky that harbors the moon, which understands the sea, from its most ferocious tempests to its darkest, coldest depths to the warmth and divine brilliance of the sun sparkling on its waves, returning us again and again to the present moment, each time delivering something new.

Acknowledgments

I offer heartfelt gratitude to Sarah Hamlin, editor at Jessica Kingsley Publishers in London, who inspired me by visualizing what the *Ocean of Yoga* could become when it was just a few waves of words. It has been a pleasure and an honor to work with her; from across the sea she has been an endless source of support, wisdom, patience, integrity, and tridoshic guidance.

A deep thank you also to the kind souls who took time and care to read various versions of my manuscript, in part or in full, and encouraged me on the path. Special thanks to Karen Dunlop, Gloria Drayer, Rosanne Lucero, Hilda Raz, Jeanne Shannon, and Cory Tixier; sincere gratitude also to Dr. Edwin G. Wilson, Dr. Tom O. Phillips, and Howard Cummins.

With endless gratefulness, I thank my family, friends, teachers, and students; I also thank the Albuquerque Bernalillo County Public Library System, the Ayurvedic Institute, Wake Forest University, music, silence, resilience, the four-legged, winged, and finned beings, and all manifestations of the five elements.

My thanks also to *The Baltimore Review*, *Janus Head*, and Finishing Line Press for granting permission for reprints of "Excavation" (*The Baltimore Review*, 2005), "The Current, the River and the Rain" (Janus Head, 2011), and "Facets," "Interwoven," "Geology of Breath" (*Breath, Bone, Earth, Sky* published by Finishing Line Press, 2014).

And deep gratitude, always, to "M" (Margaret),
whose sure-footed, four-footed spirit lives on.

About the Author

Originally from Virginia, Julie Dunlop has always loved visiting the ocean (and mountains). In relocating to New Mexico, she encountered the ocean of Yoga and Āyurveda, graduating from the Ayurvedic Institute as an Ayurvedic Health Practitioner with certification as an AyurYoga® teacher. The first time she heard of yoga was when listening to the thesis defense of a fellow graduate student in 2000 in creative writing; it was described that if you're doing a forward bend and can only reach your knees, it's important to accept this rather than straining to touch your toes. This philosophy resonated with her and she was led to explore further, soon beginning the practice of yoga. Similarly, when she was attending a world wellness health fair in Albuquerque in 2005, a volunteer at a booth asked if she'd like her pulse read. From there, she received a flyer that led her to a nearby lecture by Vasant Lad, which led her to the Ayurvedic Institute. Yoga and Āyurveda have been a vital part of her life ever since.

As a lifelong lover of language, her work integrates writing, yoga, and Āyurveda for harmony of body, mind, and soul. After earning a bachelor's degree in English from Wake Forest University in North Carolina and a master's degree in English/Creative Writing from the University of New Mexico, she began teaching writing, and over the past twenty years, has mentored thousands of writing students of various ages, backgrounds, and professions. Her writing has been published in a variety of journals and magazines, including *Journal of the American Medical Association*, *Ayurveda Journal of Health*, *Radiologic Technology*, *Wake Forest Magazine*, *Poet Lore*, *Appalachian Heritage*, *Cold Mountain Review*, *North Carolina Literary Review*, *bosque journal*, *The Baltimore Review*, *The Threepenny Review*,

Quiddity, Janus Head, South Dakota Review, Atlanta Review, and *New Mexico Poetry Review.* Her chapbooks of poetry include: *Breath, Bone, Earth, Sky* (Finishing Line Press, 2014), *Bending Back the Night* (Finishing Line Press, 2012), *Faces on the Metro* (Pudding House Press, 2005), and *Eleven A.M.* (co-author, Wildflower Press, 2003). Writing, yoga, and Āyurveda continue to find new pathways of integration in her work, honoring the healing that is at the center of both language and life.

Bibliography

Bachman, N. (2004) *The Language of Yoga*. Boulder, CO: Sounds True, Inc.

Bachman, N. (2010) *The Yoga Sutras* (workbook). Boulder, CO: Sounds True, Inc.

Kulkarni, N. (2006) *Yoga Sutras of Patanjali: Proper Translation and Chanting*. Pune: Akshar Seva.

Lad, V. (2002) *Textbook of Ayurveda, Volume 1: Fundamental Principles*. Albuquerque, NM: The Ayurvedic Press.

Lad, V. (2006) *Textbook of Ayurveda, Volume 2: A Complete Guide to Clinical Assessment*. Albuquerque, NM: The Ayurvedic Press.

Lad, V. (2012) *Textbook of Ayurveda, Volume 3: General Principles of Management and Treatment*. Albuquerque, NM: The Ayurvedic Press.

Lad, V. and Durve, A. (2008) *Marma Points of Ayurveda: The Energy Pathways for Healing Body, Mind, and Consciousness with a Comparison to Traditional Chinese Medicine*. Albuquerque, NM: The Ayurvedic Press.

Lad, V. and Garre, M. (2014) *Ayuryoga: VPK Basics*. Albuquerque, NM: The Ayurvedic Press.

Related Resources

Ayurvedic Institute (n.d.) Available at www.ayurveda.com

Banyan Botancials (n.d.) Available at https://www.banyanbotanicals.com

Davis, J. (2008) *The Journey from the Center to the Page: Yoga Philosophies and Practices as Muse for Authentic Writing*. New York: Monkfish (Original work published in 2005 by Gotham Books).

Drayer, G. and Doherty, K. (2014) *Yoga and Grief*. Bloomington, IN: Balboa Press.

Farhi, D. (1996) *The Breathing Book: Good Health and Vitality Through Essential Breath Work*. New York: Henry Holt and Company.

Farhi, D. (2006) *Teaching Yoga: Exploring the Teacher–Student Relationship*. Berkeley, CA: Rodmell Press.

Farmer, A. and Van Kooten, V. (1997) *From Inside Out: A Yoga Notebook from the Teachings of Angela and Victor*. Denver, CO: Hands on Health.

Fondin, M. (2015) *The Wheel of Healing with Ayurveda: An Easy Guide to a Healthy Lifestyle*. Novato, CA: New World Library.

Frawley, D. (1999) *Yoga and Ayurveda: Self-Healing and Self-Realization*. Twin Lakes, WI: Lotus Press.

Frawley, D. and Kozak, S. (2001) *Yoga for Your Type: An Ayurvedic Approach to Your Asana Practice*. Twin Lakes, WI: Lotus Press.

Frawley, D. and Lad, V. (2001) *The Yoga of Herbs*. Twin Lakes, WI: Lotus Press (Original work published in 1986).

Freeman, R. (2012) *The Mirror of Yoga: Awakening the Intelligence of Body and Mind*. Boston, MA: Shambhala.

Gates, J. (2006) *Yogini: The Power of Women in Yoga*. San Rafael, CA: Mandala Publishing.

Houston, V. (2002) *Bīja Mantra Chakra Tuning* (Audio CD). Collingswood, NJ: American Sanskrit Institute.

Iyengar, B.K.S. (1988) *The Tree of Yoga*. Boston, MA: Shambhala Publications.

Kabat-Zinn, J. (2013) *Full Catastrophe Living: Using the Wisdom of Your Body and Mind to Face Stress, Pain, and Illness*. New York: Bantam Books (Original work published in 1990).

Kaiminoff, L. and Matthews, A. (2012) *Yoga Anatomy*. Champaign, IL: Human Kinetics (Original work published in 2007).

Kirk, M., Boon, B., and DiTuro, D. (2006) *Hatha Yoga Illustrated*. Champaign, IL: Human Kinetics (Original work published in 2004).

Kraftsow, G. (1999) *Yoga for Wellness: Healing with the Timeless Teachings of Viniyoga*. New York: Penguin.

Lad, V. (1988) *The Complete Book of Ayurvedic Home Remedies*. New York: Three Rivers Press.

Lad, V. (2004) *Strands of Eternity*. Albuquerque, NM: The Ayurvedic Press.

Lad, V. (2006) *Secrets of the Pulse: The Ancient Art of Ayurvedic Pulse Diagnosis*. Albuquerque, NM: The Ayurvedic Press (Original work published in 1996).

Lad, V. (2009) *Ayurveda: The Science of Self-Healing*. Twin Lakes, WI: Lotus Press (Original work published in 2004).

Lad, V. (2009) *Pranayama for Self-Healing* (DVD). Albuquerque, NM: The Ayurvedic Press.

Lad, V. (2012) *Ayurvedic Perspectives on Selected Pathologies*. Albuquerque, NM: The Ayurvedic Press (Original work published in 2005).

Lad, V. and Lad, U. (2006) *Ayurvedic Cooking for Self-Healing*. Albuquerque, NM: The Ayurvedic Press (Original work published in 1994).

Little, T. (2016) *Yoga of the Subtle Body: A Guide to the Physical and Energetic Anatomy of Yoga*. Boulder, CO: Shambhala Publications.

McCall, T. (2007) *Yoga as Medicine: The Yogic Prescription for Health and Healing*. New York: Bantam Books.

Morningstar, A. (1995) *Ayurvedic Cooking for Westerners*. Twin Lakes, WI: Lotus Press.

National Ayurvedic Medical Association (n.d.) Available at www.ayurvedanama.org

NurrieStearns, M. and NurrieStearns, R. (2013) *Yoga for Emotional Trauma: Meditations and Practices for Healing Pain and Suffering*. Oakland, CA: New Harbinger Publications, Inc.

Oman, M. (1997) *Prayers for Healing: 365 Blessings, Poems, and Meditations from Around the World*. San Francisco, CA: Conari Press.

Pole, S. (2013) *Ayurvedic Medicine: The Principles of Traditional Practice*. London: Singing Dragon.

Raman, K. (1998) *A Matter of Health: Integration of Yoga and Western Medicine for Prevention and Cure*. Chennai: Eastwest Books.

Satchidananda, S. (1987) *The Golden Present: Daily Inspirational Readings*. Buckingham, VA: Integral Yoga Publications.

Shunya, A. (2017) *Ayurveda Lifestyle Wisdom: A Complete Prescription to Optimize Your Health, Prevent Disease, and Live with Vitality and Joy*. Boulder, CO: Sounds True.

Svoboda, R. (2000) *Ayurveda for Women: A Guide to Vitality and Health*. Rochester, VT: Healing Arts Press (Original work published in 1999).

Tiwari, M. (2000) *The Path of Practice: A Woman's Book of Ayurvedic Healing*. New York: Random House.

Vidal, M. (2017) *Sun, Moon, and Earth: The Sacred Relationship of Yoga and Ayurveda*. Twin Lakes, WI: Lotus Press.

Yoga Simple and Sacred (n.d.) Available at www.yogasimpleandsacred.com

Ancient Ayurvedic Texts (Translated into English)

Caraka. *Caraka Saṃhitā*. Varanasi: Chowkhamba Sanskrit Series Office, Trans. by Sharma, R.K. and Dash, B.

Mādhavakara. *Mādhava Nidānam*. Varanasi: Chaukhambha Orientalia, Trans. by Murthy, K.R.S.

Sārṅgahara. *Sārṅgahara Saṃhitā*. Varanasi: Chaukhambha Orientalia, Trans. by Murthy, K.R.S.

Suśrut. *Suśruta Saṃhitā*. Varanasi: Chaukhambha Orientalia, Trans. by Murthy, K.R.S.

Vāgbhaṭ. *Aṣṭāṅga Hṛdayam*. Varanasi: Chowkhamba Krishnadas Academy, Trans. by Murthy, K.R.S.

ॐ Namaste

May this book flow from one heart to another in our shared practice, in many styles, from many generations, in many locations, our feet rooting into the floor, our bodies coming into alignment, breathing into the moment; the mind, spirit, and body uniting, synchronizing, as we—travelers, truck drivers, dancers, business owners, magicians, morticians, accountants, soldiers, taxi drivers, computer programmers, hairstylists, biologists, chefs, waitresses, lawyers, nurses, artists, clergy, dentists, police officers, coaches, mechanics, jewelers, physicians, gardeners, sanitation workers, pilots, lifeguards, architects, toll booth collectors, farmers, librarians, social workers, lobbyists, mail carriers, daycare workers, customer service agents, psychologists, athletes, emergency medical personnel, political leaders, receptionists, philosophers, construction workers, government workers, laboratory scientists, teachers, students, musicians, cashiers, car wash attendants, reporters, veterinarians, entertainers, engineers, dreamers and doers of all kinds— as we, embracing one breath, one step, one moment at a time, become, with each ebb and flow of each cycle of our life, the ocean of yoga, with its varying tides, reflecting the light of awareness and the grace of the moon.

ॐ